Redefining Age

Modern Menopause, Naturally

ROSLYN ROGERS, CNC, BCIM

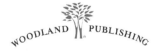

WOODLAND PUBLISHING

For permissions, ordering information, or bulk quantity discounts, contact: Woodland Publishing, Salt Lake City, UT

Visit our website: www.woodlandpublishing.com
Toll-free number (800) 777-BOOK

Note: The information in this book is for educational purposes only and is not recommended as a means of diagnosing or treating an illness. All matters concerning physical and mental health should be supervised by a health practitioner knowledgeable in treating that particular condition. Neither the publisher nor the authors directly or indirectly dispense medical advice, nor do they prescribe any remedies or assume any responsibility for those who choose to treat themselves.

ISBN 978-1-58054-213-5

Printed in the United States of America

This book is dedicated to my son Neal, who taught me so much about appreciating life and what courage is really about—to be afraid and do it anyway!

Contents

Preface

This is a good book! I am not saying that because I wrote it, but because if you accept and implement the information on each page, it will change your life and bring you better health and more joy than you can imagine.

I am not a doctor. I am only the messenger. My goal is simply to provide the steps that I have learned over the last 25 years about how to add quality years to your life, and quality life to your years!

My sincere thanks to all the medical doctors who conducted the research in this booklet, and to the naturopaths who have studied the clinical results detailed herein.

I owe a special debt of gratitude to Dr. John R. Lee, M.D., Dr. Jonathan V. Wright, M.D. and the countless healthcare practitioners who have devoted their lives to optimum health. They have all worked tirelessly to ensure that YOU can achieve better health, naturally!

And special thanks must also go to the hundreds of men and women that I have been privileged to meet in my travels. Each one of you has taught me more than I have taught you.

Roslyn Rogers

Begin the Beginning

It is time for a lifestyle change! Life is not happening to you, it is responding to you. Although good health may be your birthright, it is still a personal decision that you may need to make a thousand times each day. It's worth it! Feeling good makes life truly enjoyable.

Albert Einstein is credited with saying, "I must be willing to give up what I am in order to become what I will be." This statement certainly applies when adopting a healthier lifestyle, because we must be willing to give up habits that no longer serve us, and replace them with positive ones.

Change is not always easy. The unknown can be frightening. But in order to change unhealthy habits (such as being overweight and other behaviors that increase your risk for disease, feeling sick or generally being out of balance) you have to create new habits. So, if you have behaviors you would like to change, you need to be willing to say goodbye to them so that you can embrace the positive qualities that are better for you and your health.

Life is short, so stop procrastinating. Just do it! Today, begin whatever healthy habit you have been putting off implementing in your life. Promise yourself that you will give up one bad habit every week—following that pattern, you can eliminate 52 bad habits in one year. Now THAT is powerful!

Be Your Own Best Friend

Think for a moment about how you treat your best friend. When your best friend comes to you with a problem, you embrace her or him. If your best friend makes a mistake, you forgive him or her. We often get irritated and angry with ourselves and punish ourselves by overeating, by gaining weight, by not living in the moment and by not enjoying life. You are probably much nicer to your best friend than you are to yourself. Becoming your own best friend is a rewarding goal to pursue.

Live in the Moment

It may initially seem counterproductive, but in order to begin to change, you must accept who and what you are right now! Only when you accept yourself can you progress to the next step. Not accepting yourself for who you are can lead to frustration and anger—two emotions that contribute to bad behavior. If you are overweight, for example, it's very important to look your best, wear pretty clothes, like yourself and be your own best friend. You cannot do this without accepting who and where you are at this very moment.

Life is not about big trips or major events. Life is about the moment-to-moment occurrences that happen every single day. This is what composes your life. So, live in the moment and enjoy!

Be Proud of Your Age

As I lecture around the United States, I find myself interacting with women who have "given up" or stopped trying to change because they are over age 60. The attitude you have about your age determines whether or not you feel good. If you stop trying because you think you are too old, you will not feel very good! Loving whatever age you are is the only way to inner peace and happiness.

With age comes wisdom. If you do not feel good about your age, you will miss many of life's valuable lessons! Experiencing life is the only way to attain wisdom. All the education in the world cannot teach you what the simple act of living your life will reveal. Growing older is inevitable, but declining with age is not!

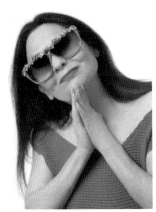

I believe a good attitude toward aging can make a huge difference in how you feel.

The phase of life after menopause is magnificent because we often do not have the same responsibilities that we did when we were younger. There are fewer demands and less stress. Accept your age and be happy. Attitude is everything. Personally, I love getting older—you can "get away" with a lot more! So, tilt your head and smile. Smiling takes 10 years off of your face.

Make the Change—Take Back your Health

Changing your habits is not about willpower. Willpower does not work because willpower does not last forever. Instead, change your habits and create new thoughts and rituals. Create a routine that you want to maintain, whether it is giving up sugar or exercising, and then maintain it for three months. After that, it becomes part of your life and is much easier to do. For example, you probably have a regular practice of brushing your teeth each morning and night. Brushing your teeth is just something that you do, because in the past, you made it a habit.

Remember, Rome was not built in a day! That is why it is important to be your own best friend—so if you take two steps forward and one step backward, do not beat yourself up. In time you will reap the rewards of the efforts you have put forward. Your health is your responsibility, not the doctor's or the pharmacist's.

Problems We Face

In the U.S., we face epidemics of breast cancer, osteoporosis, diabetes and arthritis. Such diseases now affect an entirely different group of people than they previously affected. Years ago, mostly "older" women developed breast cancer and osteoporosis. Today, breast cancer frequently strikes women in their 30s, 40s and 50s, and 50 percent of women have already begun to lose bone density by the time they reach menopause.

The major causes of disease and aging are *free radicals.* A free radical is an atom with unpaired electrons that becomes unstable when it comes in contact with oxygen. Because electrons "want" to be paired, they constantly search for another electron to create a stable pair. To become paired, free radicals "steal" electrons from other atoms. When a free radical takes an electron from an atom in the body, it creates another free radical, resulting in a continuous chain of free radical regeneration. If a free radical can't find an electron to steal, it moves around erratically in the body, damaging other cells as it comes into contact with them. When a free radical damages a cell, it causes the cell to die. This process accelerates aging and may play a role in heart disease, cancer and other diseases. Free radicals are created as a result of normal chemical reations involved in energy production, breathing and digestion as well as exposure to environmental pollutants.

Many people also consistently experience high levels of stress, which can also cause many diseases. Stress affects the adrenal glands and can weaken the immune system. It also contributes to heart disease, depression and sleep problems.

As I travel around the country speaking with women, I have found that there is a dearth of information about hormones, disease and aging. Diseases such as arthritis, high blood pressure, diabetes and heart disease are avoidable. You can make simple changes to claim your birthright of health and happiness and turn back the clock of aging. In fact, give that clock a kick!

Menopause Without Pausing

One important topic in anti-aging is hormone balance. At any age, hormones regulate many different metabolic pathways, helping you look younger and feel more energetic. The correct balance of hormones can help ward off depression, improve sleep and keep the body in a more youthful state as you age. Hormones can also help you stay active and disease-free. Your body is your own best book of health—so learn how to read it and pay attention to what it says. The goal is to die young—but as late in life as possible! One key way to accomplish this is to balance your hormones naturally.

Much of the following information is based on the writings of Dr. John R. Lee M.D., who wrote three books: *What Your Doctor May Not Tell You About Premenopause*, *What Your Doctor May Not Tell You About Menopause* and *What Your Doctor May Not Tell You About Breast Cancer*. Dr. Lee was a pioneer for information regarding the importance of using natural progesterone cream. The research that he conducted more than 20 years ago on balancing hormones naturally using natural progesterone cream is still considered extremely beneficial. So start spreading that cream!

Meet Your Hormones

In order to understand how to balance hormones naturally, it is necessary to understand a little about hormones and why they need to be balanced in the first place. Hormones are important chemical messengers in the body no matter your age. A hormone is a chemical produced by certain tissues in the body that carries information from one group of cells to another through body fluids; almost the way notes in a beautiful melody just flow.

The portion of the cell that receives these chemical signals is called a *receptor*. Each receptor site only accepts certain kinds of hormones—a receptor site is like a lock and hormones are like the key that fits right into the lock. When the hormone enters the receptor site, it signals the cell to act—to divide, or allow certain molecules to enter or exit the cell.

Hormones rule over the *endocrine system*, which regulates the thyroid, adrenal, pituitary and hypothalamus glands. Hormones play a wide variety of roles in the body—different hormones regulate growth, metabolism, tissue function and sexual function. They also play a role in determining moods. For our discussion, we will be focusing on the main sex hormones in women, *estrogen* and *progesterone*, as well as *testosterone*, which is often considered the male hormone, but is also found in women.

Estrogen is the primary sex hormone in women of childbearing age. It is produced in the ovaries, adrenal glands and fat. Estrogen plays an important role in the growth and development of female sexual characteristics and in reproduction. Estrogen also works with calcium and vitamin D to build bones and prevent bone loss.

Progesterone is another one of the sex hormones. However, progesterone is slightly different from other sex hormones such as estrogen and testosterone. As discussed, estrogen is important for the growth and development of female sexual characteristics. Similarly, testosterone is a hormone responsible for proper development of male sexual characteristics (although women need a little testosterone, too). In contrast, progesterone does not provide any sexual characteristics. Both male and female babies bathe in progesterone for nine months during gestation. During her last trimester of pregnancy, a woman produces between 300–400 mg of progesterone each day. (Normally, a menstruating woman makes about 20–24 mg of progesterone each day.)

The large amount of progesterone produced during pregnancy produces the beautiful "glow" common to pregnant women. It is also considered "the feel good hormone." Progesterone helps convert fat into energy, helps to metabolize glucose (the simple sugar that functions as the body's main energy source), stimulates bone formation, restores libido, works as a natural diuretic, calms anxiety and much more. It also works as a building block for other hormones in the body, such as cortisol (which helps regulate the body's use of energy), testosterone and estrogen. Progesterone is also important for the health of the myelin sheath, the insulating layer around nerves of the spine. When the body does not have sufficient progesterone, it can cause pain and aching in the spine.

PERIMENOPAUSE AND MENOPAUSE—STEPS TO WISDOM?

Stop thinking that menopause is synonymous to old age! At a certain age, every woman must go through a time when she no longer has a menstrual cycle and cannot conceive a child. That time is often a great occurrence as we can now enjoy sex without the worry of becoming pregnant. Many cultures around the world praise this time, when women can concentrate on themselves. Among the Maya in rural Guatemala and the Yucatán peninsula in Mexico, many women look forward to menopause because of the increase in social status and freedom it brings. After menopause, they are known as "wise women" and gain a place of power in their communities. Women in India enjoy a similar increase in social status.

Consider menopause a happy step in your life's continuing journey.

I also love the attitude in northern Sudan, where menopause is regarded as simply an aspect of growing older—bringing with it increased social power and respect. For many women around the world, menopause means that children have grown up and her daily duties to family life have eased off. Like the Sudanese, I suggest thinking of menopause as just another step in the continuing journey of life.

However, if you don't feel well during this time, is it certainly harder to climb those steps. And that is where balancing hormones can play a very important role in how you feel and how you enjoy each day.

Women typically experience symptoms of menopause in different stages. The first stage is *premenopause*, the portion of a woman's life between her first menstrual period and her last regular menstrual period. Premenopause is followed by *perimenopause*, a time of transition that usually lasts between two and 10 years. Women are usually between 35 and 50 years of age when they enter perimenopause. The perimenopause stage is characterized by what are usually thought of as menopausal symptoms: hormonal fluctuations, hot flashes, mood swings and vaginal dryness. During this time, a woman's menstrual cycle is irregular. Perimenopause ends when a woman experiences her final menstrual period.

A woman reaches *menopause* 12 months after her final menstrual period. After this point, called *postmenopause*, menopause symptoms typically decrease, although post-menopausal women are at an increased risk for certain diseases, including osteoporosis and heart disease. Just because a woman is postmenopausal does not mean that she cannot stay in hormonal balance. The opposite is true— hormonal balance is especially important for health at this time of life.

Hormone levels naturally fluctuate during peri-menopause and menopause. Even when a woman no longer menstruates, her body still makes estrogen. When a woman's ovaries stop producing eggs and the hormone estrogen, the adrenal glands take over estrogen production so that estrogen levels only decrease about 40–50 percent compared with estrogen levels prior to menopause. After menopause, the adrenal glands continue to make estrogen for a woman's entire life. However, production of progesterone decreases dramatically following menopause, which can lead to hormone imbalance.

Too Much of a Good Thing

A woman once asked me an interesting question following one of my lectures about balancing hormones naturally. She asked, "If menopause is such a natural occurrence, why do we have to do anything about it?"

She is correct. Menopause *is* a natural occurrence, not a disease (as is often the attitude today). However, due to changes in the way we have lived over the past 100 years, with the many toxins in the environment, many menopausal women experience symptoms that can disrupt their lives—including difficulty sleeping, memory problems and hot flashes.

Many of the symptoms menopausal women experience stem from a hormonal imbalance due to *estrogen dominance*. While estrogen plays many important roles in the body, the body needs progesterone to oppose and balance it. When the body has too much estrogen and not enough progesterone to oppose it, the result is estrogen dominance. Estrogen dominance is determined by the body's levels of estrogen compared to levels of progesterone. Such a condition can occur in women who have very low estrogen levels, if levels of progesterone are even lower.

An imbalance of estrogen and progesterone can cause a variety of problems in the body—including increasing symptoms of menopause. Often estrogen dominance is associated with breast and uterine cancer in women and prostate cancer in men.

Estrogen Dominance Symptoms:

- hot flashes
- night sweats
- weight gain—(especially under the breasts and around the waist)
- thyroid problems (fatigue, constipation, poor tolerance to cold, insomnia and nervousness) *See page 37 for more information*
- fibrocystic breasts (a benign condition in which the breasts are composed of tissue that feels lumpy, ropy or bumpy)
- fibroid tumors (benign tumors in the uterus, usually found in women in their 30s and 40s)
- "foggy" brain (memory and cognitive problems)
- endometriosis (a condition in which cells from the uterus lining grow outside the uterine cavity, causing pelvic pain and bleeding)
- water retention
- sleeplessness
- loss of libido
- vaginal dryness
- infertility

According to Dr. Lee's research, estrogen dominance is common because of the industrialized world. Much of what we use on a daily basis is made from *petroleum*, or crude oil, a naturally-occurring flammable liquid used to make products ranging from gasoline to cosmetics. Petroleum contains estrogen-imitating toxins called *xenoestrogens*. Such byproducts of petroleum can behave like estrogens in the body and have strong and harmful effects.

Xenoestrogens enter breast and uterine hormone receptor sites and mimic estrogen, creating diseases and hormonal imbalances with very uncomfortable symptoms. The body cannot tell the difference between naturally-produced estrogen and estrogen imitators from the environment—they both fit the same receptor sites. However, the estrogen produced by the body behaves differently than petroleum-derived estrogen imitators. Hormones produced by the body are made naturally, utilized as needed and then eliminated. In contrast, xenoestrogens are stored in fatty tissues, potentially causing a lot of problems.

Petroleum is used to make clothing, and is found in shampoos, hair conditioners, body lotions, fertilizers, ordinary household cleansers, dryer fabric softeners, plastic bottles and fragrances from candles and perfumes. Toxic chemicals from petroleum are found in the air we breathe, the food we eat and the water we drink. They are everywhere! It is almost impossible not to come in contact with environmental toxins from petroleum.

Preservatives in food are another potential danger. Growing your own food used to be the norm in an agricultural society. Now, people who grow their own food are definitely in the minority. Many people subsist on a steady diet of processed food loaded with preservatives. Manufacturers add preservatives to food to increase shelf life and enhance flavor—but what do preservatives do to the body? Mounting evidence suggests that preservatives may have dangerous effects. For example, one class of preservative found in food, cosmetics and pharmaceuticals are *parabens,* which are xenoestrogens.

Another cause of extra estrogen in the body is estrogen found in meat. Estrogen is often given to cattle and other animals (in the form of small pellets placed behind the animal's ear) because it causes livestock to gain water weight, helping the animals grow bigger and fatter—and get to market faster. If you are eating non-organic beef and dairy products such as cheese, milk and yogurt, you are ingesting estrogen, estrogen and more estrogen.

If all that was not enough, women commonly take birth control pills and hormone replacement therapy (discussed below), which puts more estrogen into the body. Combine these factors with exposure to xenoestrogens from the environment, and it is easy to understand why it is common for women to be so out of balance and symptomatic.

HORMONE REPLACEMENT THERAPY

Hormone replacement therapy (HRT) refers to medications that contain female hormones designed to replace those that the body does not produce during and after menopause. Physicians prescribe HRT to treat symptoms of menopause, chiefly hot flashes, night sweats and vaginal dryness.

The U.S. Food and Drug Administration (FDA) approved a synthetic estrogen from horse urine to treat menopausal symptoms in 1942. Hormone replacement therapy (HRT) first became popular during the 1950s. At that time, women were beginning to feel particularly symptomatic during menopause. The prevailing conventional wisdom was "better living through chemistry." Penicillin had just been discovered and vaccines were preventing diseases and saving lives. For many people, pharmaceutical drugs were beginning to replace traditional homeopathic treatments. So pharmaceutical companies developed drugs to treat symptoms of menopause as well.

When synthetic HRT was introduced, doctors suggested that estrogen was a way to keep women healthy and sexy for years after menopause. For many years, if a woman over age 40 went to see her doctor with any complaint, she was most often given a prescription for estrogen. And taking estrogen did eliminate hot flashes and other menopausal symptoms.

But doctors soon discovered that estrogen also caused many serious complications, primarily an increased risk of uterine cancer. To lessen complications associated with estrogen therapy, doctors added progestin (a synthetic progesterone hormone). At the time, doctors claimed that taking estrogen and progestin would protect against heart disease and breast and uterine cancer. By the 1990s, a combination of estrogen and progestin had become the second most commonly-prescribed medication in the United States.

The National Institutes of Health (NIH) formed the Women's Health Initiative (WHI) in 1991 to conduct clinical trials to study major health problems in menopausal women. In 1997, the WHI began a large study designed to measure risks and benefits of HRT. Researchers selected over 16,000 women between the ages of 50 and 79 to participate in the study. Half of the participants were given a combination of estrogen and progestin and the other half received a placebo.

Researchers planned the study to last for eight years, but in 2002, after five years, the monitoring committee abruptly stopped the trials. They cited results of an independent safety monitoring board that found that the risks of the therapy were not worth the benefits. According to the results, the women in the study who took the combinations of estrogen and progestin had experienced increased incidence of several diseases, including:

- 26 percent increase in incidence of invasive breast cancer
- 29 percent increase in the risk of heart attacks
- 50 percent increase in the risk of dementia
- 50 percent increase in the risk of blood clots
- 41 percent increase in incidence of strokes

(*Source: "Facts About Menopause Hormone Therapy," a 2005 report published by the U.S. Department of Health and Human Services and the National Institutes of Health.*)

Additionally, the researchers reported that the breasts of the women taking the estrogen/progestin combination became so dense that it was difficult to properly read their mammograms.

When the WHI study stopped prematurely, many women threw away their hormone pills and doctors stopped writing HRT prescriptions as readily. However, pharmaceutical companies that produced synthetic HRT also fought back, dismissing the study results. Today, many allopathic doctors are again recommending synthetic HRT. But we do not have to take it! We can say "no!"

Surviving Hot Flashes

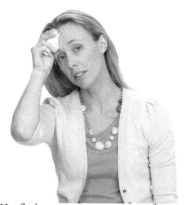

Hot flashes, a common symptom of menopause, can disrupt everyday life.

While HRT may not be the solution, that does not mean that hot flashes and other symptoms of menopause should be dismissed! Up to 80 percent of women experience hot flashes during menopause. Hot flashes can cause sleep disruptions, leading to energy, mood and cognitive function problems. They are a legitimate concern for many menopausal women.

The good news is that we do not need synthetic drugs and hormones to manage hot flashes. Taking pharmaceutical drugs to get rid of hot flashes is like using a gun to shoot a fly—it is overkill!

One easy way to survive hot flashes is to dress in lightweight clothing. Or dress in layers, so if you feel a hot flash coming on, you can cool down by removing a layer of clothing.

Hot flashes are sometimes triggered by foods. To keep track of which foods may give you trouble, try keeping a food journal. Often, if you write down what you eat and when you experience hot flashes, you can see a pattern connecting the symptoms with diet. Carbohydrates, caffeine and sugar are common triggers.

Natural Progesterone: An Alternative to HRT

Natural progesterone (derived from wild yams) is generally safe and can aid in opposing the effects of harmful environmental xenoestrogens. I have seen results that I would call miraculous in hundreds of women who use it! After using natural progesterone from wild yams, some women tell me that their hot flashes go away, they sleep better, lose weight easier, their thinking becomes clearer and hormonal headaches and PMS become a thing of their past. And natural progesterone can decrease the risk of developing breast and uterine cancer!

Progesterone derived from the wild yam plant is not a synthetic hormone. Instead, natural progesterone cream is considered a *bioidentical hormone*, which means that it is derived from plants and is chemically identical to the hormones found naturally in the body. In contrast, progestins used in pharmaceutical HRT are synthetic and not bioidentical. Like the xenoestrogens discussed earlier, synthetic hormones often get stored in the fat of the body, staying there for years and causing all kinds of imbalances and unwanted symptoms.

PROGESTERONE IN PREMENOPAUSAL WOMEN

In addition to helping to ease menopausal symptoms, progesterone cream from wild yams can be helpful for younger women who have not yet entered menopause. Younger women can have imbalanced hormones due to toxins in the environment. In such cases, the body may produce a normal amount of hormones, but still be out of balance because so much estrogen enters the body from environmental sources.

Younger women should consider progesterone on an individual basis. Consult with a healthcare practitioner before using progesterone cream. He or she can perform a urine or saliva test to check progesterone levels.

Hormonal imbalance may contribute to:

- polycystic ovarian syndrome (PCOS)
- severe premenstrual syndrome (PMS)
- cysts in breasts
- irregular menstrual cycles
- infertility (if the body does not have enough progesterone, it is difficult to conceive or "hold" a baby, so miscarriage is common)
- menstrual cramping
- hormonal headaches

USING NATURAL PROGESTERONE CREAM

The most effective way to use natural progesterone is through transdermal application. Transdermal application means that progesterone is applied and absorbed through the skin. Applying progesterone transdermally is one of the best ways to quickly get hormones directly into the system. When you apply a cream to the skin, it immediately enters the system, bypassing stomach acids and enzymes that can destroy its potency. Very little progesterone affects the liver, which has a hard time processing large doses of oral hormones. Transdermal rather than oral progesterone also minimizes stomach upset, a common occurrence when taking hormones orally. Transdermal application is a proven, effective delivery system to introduce progesterone directly into the bloodstream.

How can you use transdermal progesterone cream? Women who are no longer menstruating should use progesterone for three weeks and take one week off each month. Women who are still menstruating should use progesterone in conjunction with their natural cycles. Begin using progesterone 12 days after the first day of the period (considered "day one" of the menstrual cycle) and continue until the 26th day of the cycle.

Although not all progesterone creams come in pumps, the easiest way to get the correct dose is to use a cream that dispenses 20 mg of progesterone per pump (in keeping with the normal amount that women make in their ovaries). When purchasing progesterone cream, be sure to check the label. Purchase only all natural United States Pharmacopoeia (USP) grade progesterone with no parabens.

Progesterone can be used once or twice daily on parts of the body with thinner skin—the best places are wrists, chest, inner arms and legs, neck and stomach area. To avoid saturating one area, rotate and use the cream on different parts of the body each day. Sing while you apply.

Wake Up the Vagina

Let's talk about libido. Everyone is born with libido. For women, libido is not necessarily all about having sex. It can be about motivation and wanting to be active, vibrant and present. Libido in women is related to happiness, feeling good and general well-being. It has a lot to do with caring about one's self, having better energy and endurance and being able to live life to the fullest. Having a good libido is a wonderful motivator. And of course, that includes having a fulfilling sex life!

Of course we all want to feel good! So how can you boost your libido and wake up your vagina? Start by throwing out any worn underwear with holes in it! Then try the following tips.

USE TESTOSTERONE-BUILDING SUPPLEMENTAL CREAMS

Although many people think that testosterone is only for men, women sometimes need help with libido. While women need about one-tenth testosterone that men need, they do need some. This is especially true with the current toxic environment. Estrogen dominance affects testosterone as well. Chemicals in foods can destroy natural hormones, including testosterone, contributing to estrogen dominance.

Like progesterone creams, testosterone creams can be applied transdermally. It is easiest to use a cream in a pre-measured pump. Look for testosterone creams made with herbal bioidentical hormones. Herbs such as catuaba (*Erythroxylum catuaba*), which comes from the bark of a tree found in northern Brazil, and shatavari root (*Asparagus racemosus*), a species of asparagus found in Sri Lanka, India and the Himalayas, have been used to boost libido for centuries.

Try Some Kegel Exercises!

Named for the California gynecologist who "invented" them, Kegel exercises help strengthen the pelvic floor muscles (the muscles that support the uterus, bladder and bowels). The pelvic floor muscles are important for bladder control and for sexual satisfaction and orgasm. Women's pelvic floor muscles are often weakened by pregnancy and childbirth, being overweight and aging.

To learn which muscles to contract to complete a "Kegel," try to stop the flow of your urine while urinating. That is the basic "move" of a Kegel exercise. Once you know which muscles to contract, empty your bladder, sit or lie down and contract the pelvic floor muscles. Hold for five seconds, then relax for five seconds. Repeat this 8–10 times three times throughout the day. Work up to contracting the muscles for 10 seconds and relaxing for 10 seconds.

Make sure that you keep your abdominal, thigh and buttock muscles relaxed while completing Kegel exercises. Otherwise, you will not be exercising the right muscles and you will not see the benefits! You may need to perform Kegel exercises regularly for up to 12 weeks before you notice a difference. But what's 12 weeks of exercise if you can wake up from sexual hibernation?

Use Estriol Cream Vaginally

One common symptom of menopause is vaginal dryness, which can make sex painful and unenjoyable. Estriol, the weakest of the three main forms of estrogen that the body produces, can help with these symptoms. Since estriol is lower potency than estradiol and estrione, the other forms of estrogen, it does not increase the risk of hormone-dependent cancers like the other forms of estrogen. Studies indicate that topically applying estriol cream vaginally can help alleviate vaginal dryness. When applied topically and locally, estriol can help alleviate vaginal dryness.

Brownies By Maca

My favorite libido boosting supplement is maca. Maca is a cruciferous root vegetable that Peruvians have used for centuries for libido, energy, fertility and sexual pleasure. Healthcare practitioners often recommend maca in place of HRT. Maca may help with mood, anxiety and depression problems in postmenopausal women.

Recent research supports the idea that maca may help alleviate some menopausal symptoms and increase libido. In a 2008 study published in the journal *Menopause*, researchers studied a small group of postmenopausal women. Half of the women received 3.5 g of powdered maca daily for six weeks, while the other half received a placebo. The groups then switched. While their blood samples of hormone concentrations were not significantly different over the 12-week study period, the women's scores on the Greene Climacteric Scale, which assesses the severity of menopausal symptoms, did change significantly. While taking maca powder, the women's psychological menopausal symptoms, particularly anxiety and depression, decreased, as did measures of sexual dysfunction.

Maca does not contain any hormones. Instead, it is an adaptogen, a type of herb that helps balance hormone production by helping the body produce whatever hormones it lacks. Maca contains large amounts of amino acids, carbohydrates and minerals that stimulate hormone production. For this reason, maca is wonderful for both men and women.

Although maca is available in liquid or capsule form, in my experience, it absorbs better in the body in a powdered form. Maca powder may be added to juice or water. Peruvians use maca powder to make cookies, cakes, hot porridge and chips.

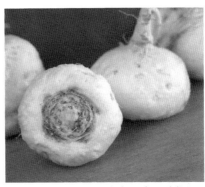

Add maca root to your baking for a delicious way to boost libido!

You can even have a party and serve maca brownies! But I am not responsible for anyone's behavior after eating.

(*Note: Since maca may stimulate the central nervous system, do not use maca if you have high blood pressure.*)

Becoming Balanced, Naturally

Calm, Cool, Collected

These days, stress levels are high. Do you know anybody who is not stressed? Although stress is a part of life, studies show that many diseases are related to stress on the immune system. Stress can be especially damaging to the adrenal and thyroid glands. Hormones rule both the thyroid and adrenal glands. Managing stress and keeping hormones in balance can help these vital glands work properly.

ADRENALS

When you encounter a stressful situation, your body has a number of physical and psychological responses. One of the body's chief responses to stress is stimulating the adrenal glands—small glands located above the kidneys. When the body is under stress, the adrenal glands produce hormones in response. One of the body's primary stress hormones is *cortisol*, which provides a quick energy boost and lowers pain sensitivity, but also increases blood pressure and impairs the immune system.

Another stress hormone is *adrenaline*, which is a neurotransmitter (a chemical that transmits information from one cell to another) that increases heart rate and constricts the blood vessels to prepare the body for a "fight or flight" response. When cortisol and adrenaline are released, the muscles become tense and the body diverts energy away from long-term uses, such as tissue repair, focusing energy in the muscles. The immune system is inhibited so the body can focus on the source of the stress.

In the short term, the stress response is helpful as it can serve as a motivator and help you get through dangerous or challenging situations. However, many sources of stress are a constant, chronic part of life, rather than a fleeting situation that requires a quick burst of hormones and muscle strength.

As a result of constant stress, the body repeatedly signals the adrenal glands to produce cortisol. While short-term cortisol production is good for the body, chronic stress and constant production of cortisol can lead to damage to the tissues and increase the risk of disease. Chronic stress leads to difficulty sleeping and overproduction of cortisol can also cause problems with weight management. If the adrenal glands secrete too much cortisol, the body may respond as if it is going into "starvation mode" and stop metabolizing and burning fat.

Ultimately, the adrenal glands can become exhausted to the point that they can no longer produce sufficient cortisol. This condition, known as *adrenal fatigue*, can cause a variety of symptoms, including profound fatigue and weakened muscles.

THYROID

The thyroid gland, located in the neck, plays an important role in almost every metabolic process in the body. It produces hormones, including triiodothyronine (T_3), which helps control growth, development, metabolism, body temperature and heart rate; and thyroxine (T_4), which influences physical development. The thyroid also controls how quickly the body uses energy.

The most common problems related to the thyroid involve abnormal production of thyroid hormones. When the thyroid underproduces hormones, hypothyroidism results. When the thyroid overproduces hormones, hyperthyroidism results. Both hypo- and hyperthyroidism upset the chemical balance of the body and can cause fatigue and depression. Anxiety attacks can also be related to thyroid imbalances.

As I travel around the country, a very high percentage of the women I meet have either been diagnosed with thyroid problems, or think they may have thyroid problems but their blood tests do not show an imbalance.

In my opinion, the blood test for thyroid is not always effective. It may only show major thyroid imbalances and does not necessarily detect if the thyroid is "off" just a little bit. But even if the thyroid is only under- or overproducing hormones by a small amount, it can make a huge difference in how you feel.

Women over the age of 50 are more likely to suffer from hypothyroidism. Symptoms can include irritability, sleeplessness, weight gain, brittle hair, joint pain and cold sensitivity. Such symptoms typically develop gradually over a period of years.

A variety of factors can lead to developing hypothyroidism, but one main cause is a lack of iodine in the diet. Without iodine, the thyroid cannot produce hormones. Iodine is found in seafood, seaweed, plants grown in iodine-rich soil and iodized salt. Years ago, salt producers began adding iodine to salt to combat a widespread iodine deficiency. However, in recent years many individuals have begun using less salt, as salt intake became associated with obesity, high blood pressure and heart disease. Consequently, iodine intake also decreased.

In addition, certain minerals commonly found in tap water can inhibit the body's absorption of iodine. Fluoride (commonly added to water to prevent tooth decay) and bromine and chlorine (used to disinfect water) are the main culprits. All four of these elements compete for absorption in the body. Because fluoride, chloride and bromine are all lighter than iodine, they easily displace iodine when they are present, leading to an iodine deficiency.

WAYS TO BECOME CALM, COOL AND COLLECTED

Chemical-laden diets, insufficient amounts of vitamins and minerals and "couch potatoism" all contribute to inner turmoil and imbalances. However, ancient but effective ways to combat stress and heal the thyroid and adrenal glands exist.

Learning stress management techniques may be the most important way to reduce the damaging effects of stress. You've heard it before . . . start by getting sufficient sleep and exercise! Meditation, yoga and taking time to relax can also reduce the impact of stress.

Breathing is a wonderful way to relax the entire body. Deep breathing sends a message to the brain to calm down and relax. Physical effects of stress, including increased heart rate, rapid breathing and high blood pressure, decrease when you breathe deeply to relax. While deep breathing exercises can be incredibly relaxing, it also fills the cells of your body with more oxygen, which can be very energizing.

Most of us do not take advantage of the incredible health benefits of deep breathing. Here are some ways to begin:

Sit quietly and close your eyes. Take a deep breath while counting to five, filling your ribcage with air and continuing to take in air all the way up to your chest. When you can't take in any more air, hold your breath for five seconds. Exhale for five seconds and when you think all your air is out, puff out just a little more. Continue this exercise for five minutes, and gradually increase in length until you set aside 15 minutes

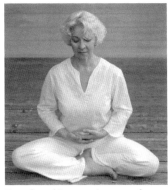

Deep breathing exercises can relax the body.

in the morning and 15 minutes at night to do your deep breathing exercises.

Another technique that I like, especially when I am finding it hard to sit and relax, is called "alternate nostril breathing." In order to do this breathing exercise, you need to concentrate, which takes your mind off your moment of stress.

Begin by sitting quietly and placing your thumb on one side of your nose and your middle finger on the other side. Gently take your thumb away from one nostril and exhale out. Then breathe in from the same nostril and put your thumb back and hold for a few seconds. Next exhale by removing your middle finger from the other nostril and then breathing in more air from that same side. Place both fingers over your nose and hold for a couple of seconds. Continue for 5–10 minutes, alternating breathing through each nostril.

HERBAL SUPPORT—LET THE SUNSHINE IN!

In addition to deep breathing, *adaptogenic herbs* can be very beneficial for relaxation. As their name suggests, adaptogens help the body adapt to and deal with the effects of stress. An adaptogenic herb helps strengthen the body's response against physical, chemical or biological stressors by recharging the adrenal glands. Adaptogens help the body handle stress and relieve fatigue, while causing minimal disruption to the body. Some of my favorite adaptogens include:

Ashwagandha. This shrub is native to India, Sri Lanka and Pakistan. It plays an important role in Ayurvedic medicine, a traditional system of medicine that originated in India. Ashwagandha is a mild sedative with a calming effect. Ayurvedic practitioners have used ashwagandha for centuries to treat stress and relieve anxiety.

Rhodiola. A small plant with yellow flowers, *Rhodiola rosea* grows in Arctic areas in North America, Europe, Siberia and Asia. It is often used to improve mood and alleviate depression. In 2000, researchers conducted a double-blind placebo-controlled study on the effects of rhodiola in healthy individuals. The study, published in *Phytomedicine*, found that administering a low dose of rhodiola for 20 days prior to a stressful exam period improved physical fitness and mental fatigue as well as improving how individuals assessed their stress levels.

Ginseng. Cultivated in Korea and China, true ginseng, or *Panax ginseng*, has been used for over 2,000 years in traditional Chinese medicine. The root or rhizome of the ginseng plant is the most medicinally valuable part of the plant. Ginseng promotes relaxation, supports the immune system and can stimulate the central nervous system in cases of prolonged emotional stress.

L-Theanine. L-theanine was originally isolated from the *Camellia sinensis* plant, which is used to produce green and black tea. Produced synthetically, L-theanine may help relieve stress by inducing relaxation. In a study published in 2007 in *Biological Psychology*, researchers compared psychological and physiological responses of individuals in stressful situations. The researchers reported that taking L-theanine supplements either at the beginning or midway through the experimental procedure lowered heart rate and production of salivary immunoglobulin A, a major component of the body's physiological stress response. The researchers concluded that L-theanine may combat both mental and physical effects of stress.

Holy Basil. Native to India but now cultivated worldwide, holy basil (*Ocimum tenuiflorum*) is a large shrub with green or purple leaves. Like ashwagandha, holy basil plays an important role in Ayurvedic medicine. Holy basil is often used in India to treat stress-related problems. It may help reduce elevated cortisol levels.

B-Vitamins. B-complex vitamins are also excellent for helping the body deal with stress. See page 79 for more information about how B-vitamins can help you become calm, cool and collected.

Your Achy-Breaky Heart

Of all the body parts that can break, the heart is the only one that can heal itself (of course, only at an "emotional" level). But aside from the emotional pain of a broken heart, physical heart problems can pose a great threat to both your happiness and health! The Centers for Disease Control and Prevention (CDC) reports that heart disease is the number one killer of women. Women are especially at risk for heart problems after menopause.

HEART-FRIENDLY SUPPLEMENTS

Dr. Stephen T. Sinatra M.D., a board-certified cardiologist, has made amazing contributions to improving heart health. In *The Sinatra Solution: New Hope for Preventing and*

Treating Heart Disease, he writes about the importance of restoring "good energy" to the heart. The nutrients that he suggests are imperative for heart health are coenzyme Q10, L-carnitine, D-ribose and magnesium. The combination of these supplements will not only bring more oxygen to the heart for better cardiac energy, but can also increase the energy for the entire body. Who couldn't use that?

Coenzyme Q10. This vitamin-like substance is found in every cell of the body. The body produces some CoQ-10, which the cells use to produce adenosine triphosphate (ATP), the body's main source of energy. The body needs ATP for basic cell function. CoQ-10 is an important nutrient for the heart and brain, both of which require a lot of ATP to meet their high energy needs. CoQ-10 can also function as an *antioxidant*, a natural compound that helps defend the body against damage from free radicals. Remember, a free radical is unstable because it has an unpaired electron. An antioxidant is a natural compound that prevents free radical damage by sacrificing an electron to neutralize a free radical. When an antioxidant gives an electron to a free radical, the free radical is paired and becomes stable. As an antioxidant, CoQ-10 helps promote cardiovascular health, control inflammation and maintain healthy cholesterol levels.

The body's production of CoQ-10 tends to decrease with age, so supplementing the diet with CoQ-10 may be necessary to maintain proper cell function. Statin drugs, used to lower cholesterol, also lower the body's stores of CoQ-10. Anyone taking a natural or pharmaceutical statin should take a CoQ-10 supplement to balance this effect.

Foods that contain CoQ-10 include sardines, beef and peanuts, although you would need to eat eight pounds of peanuts to get a 100 mg serving (the typical recommended intake ranges between 30–200 mg of CoQ-10 per day).

L-Carnitine. The body synthesizes L-carnitine from lysine and methionine, two amino acids. Usually, the body can synthesize this important nutrient, but in some cases the body's demand for L-carnitine can exceed the body's ability to produce it.

L-carnitine may help prevent a heart attack. In 2000, researchers studied the effects of L-carnitine supplements on patients with heart failure. The study, published in the *American Heart Journal*, looked at 80 patients with moderate to severe heart failure. Half of the participants received two grams of L-carnitine while the other half received a placebo. Researchers reported that the three-year survival rate of heart failure patients receiving L-carnitine supplements was significantly higher than the placebo group.

D-Ribose. The body naturally produces D-ribose, a type of sugar. D-ribose is the building block of DNA and RNA and helps the body produce ATP. It may help rejuvenate heart muscles damaged during a heart attack and protect against cell damage that occurs during a heart attack.

A review of several studies published in 2004 in *Experimental and Clinical Cardiology* reported that in both animal and human clinical trials, D-ribose supplements had benefits for congestive heart failure (CHF). In one of the human clinical trials referenced (published in 1992 in *Lancet*), researchers gave either 60 grams of D-ribose or a placebo to 20 men with coronary heart disease. They found that the men who received the D-ribose supplement were able to exercise longer without ill effects to the heart. D-ribose may help fight the fatigue common in patients with CHF by helping the body recover ATP.

Magnesium. A diet rich in magnesium may also help protect against cardiovascular disease, according to a 2006 study published in *Circulation*. The study found that young adults ages 18–30 with higher magnesium intake were less likely to develop metabolic syndrome, a condition that increases the risk of heart disease. Magnesium helps regulate the heart's pumping action by causing the heart muscle to relax. By regulating heartbeat, magnesium helps decrease the risk of developing abnormal heart rhythms, which are associated with heart attack.

Note: Please see a healthcare practitioner before beginning this protocol, particulary if you have a history of any heart disturbances or problems.

Breast Cancer

According to the CDC, breast cancer is the most common type of cancer among women in the United States and the leading cause of cancer death among women. According to www.breastcancer.org, a nonprofit website that provides information about breast cancer, one in eight women will be diagnosed with breast cancer during her lifetime.

After my lectures, women often ask what steps they can take to help lessen their chances of getting breast cancer. This is certainly a good question. There are many things that a woman can do to stay healthy. Let's discuss a few nutrients that may be helpful in preventative medicine.

Green Tea. Brewed from minimally processed leaves from the *Camellia sinensis* plant, green tea contains catechins, a type of *phytonutrient* (a natural plant compound with health-protecting qualities). Catechins are great antioxidants. Green tea is less processed than black or oolong teas, so it retains a higher concentration of catechins.

Green tea may help inhibit cancer growth. A study conducted in Japan and published in 1998 in the *Japanese Journal of Cancer Research* studied 472 women with breast cancer. The researchers found that women who consumed more green tea experienced less cancer spread. Women who drank four or more cups per day were less likely to experience recurrence of breast cancer. Green tea can be beneficial whether taken in a cup as a tea or in supplement form. Green tea is also common as a ready-to-drink beverage.

Indole-3-Carbinol. Indole-3-carbinol, found in cruciferous vegetables such as cabbage, broccoli, Brussels sprouts and cauliflower, is another powerful phytonutrient. Compounds in indole-3-carbinol may help reverse estrogen dominance. Indole-3-carbinol may also

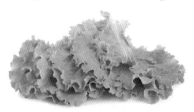

Indole-3-carbinol, from leafy green vegetables, can promote healthy hormone balance.

help the body produce more 2-hydroxyestrone (a form of estrogen that protects against cancer) and less 16-hydroxyestrone (a carcinogenic form of estrogen). In a 1997 study published in the *Journal of the National Cancer Institute*, researchers at the Strang Cancer Prevention Lab in New York City studied the effects of indole-3-carbinol supplementation. The researchers reported that in women who took a 400 mg daily dose of indole-3-carbinol, the levels of 2-hydroxyestrone were higher while 16-hydroxyestrone levels were lower.

Calcium D-Glucarate. Another nutrient that I think is wonderful is calcium D-glucarate, a detoxifying chemical. Calcium D-glucarate combines calcium with glucaric acid, a chemical found naturally in the body as well as in fruits and vegetables including grapefruits, apples, spinach, Brussels sprouts and oranges. Calcium D-glucarate can neutralize toxic free radicals.

Research shows that estrogen binds with glucaric acid in the liver, so that the estrogen can be excreted in bile instead of being reabsorbed in the bloodstream, where it can cause cell proliferation. Some women report that calcium D-glucarate eliminates hot flashes and reduces weight gain caused by estrogen dominance. Good health can begin now with this winning partnership.

Bones Are Living Tissue

Bones are living tissue that can renew, grow and mend. So, the body is capable of making new bone throughout one's life. If your nails and hair grow, your bones can grow. From birth to the age of 20 we make more bone than we lose. From ages 20 to 35 bone density peaks, then begins to steadily decline afterward. *Osteoporosis* is a progressive disease where bone loss exceeds new bone formation. Such an imbalance can result in fractures. Osteoporosis is not a disease of menopause as it begins five to 20 years before menopause.

Cells called *osteoclasts* travel through bone removing old bone and in the process leaving tiny spaces. Cells called *osteoblasts* then move in to make new and stronger bone. Long bones, such as arm and leg bones, are very dense and take 10–12 years to turn over. Bones that are less dense, like the heel and vertebrae in the spine, may have a 100 percent turnover in two to three years.

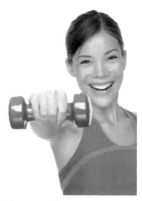

Lifting weights can help you strengthen your muscles and your bones.

To prevent osteoporosis, each individual needs to find the right balance of bone loss and bone renewal. Hydrochloric acid (HCl) is particularly important for breaking down calcium in the stomach so that it can be absorbed through the intestines. HCl can help manage osteoporosis, which happens when bones do not have sufficient calcium. Many people with osteoporosis are not calcium deficient, rather the calcium they consume is not being absorbed by the bones.

Other important nutrients for strong bones are vitamins D_3 and K_2, and minerals like calcium and magnesium, strontium and silica. While estrogen has very little to do with making new bone, it helps delay the loss of bone. Estrogen helps the bones absorb calcium and helps maintain bone density. Weight-bearing exercises are also important in maintaining bone strength. And, according to research conducted by Dr. John Lee and published in *What Your Doctor May Not Tell You About Menopause*, balancing your hormones may also help the body find the right balance between bone loss and bone renewal. Using natural progesterone in a transdermal cream may be helpful. As the famous Chinese philosopher Lao Tzu (604–531 B.C.) wrote, "a journey of a thousand miles begins with a single step."

The Art of Beautiful Skin

The skin needs the proper nutrients inside and out. The ingredients that you apply on your skin topically are just as important as the ingredients you ingest. The following nutrients can help promote beautiful skin.

INSIDE OUT

Beautiful skin begins on the inside. When the body has sufficient supplies of the proper nutrients, beautiful skin naturally results. Try the following tips to build beautiful skin from the inside out:

Drink Up! Water is one of the skin's basic needs. Drinking sufficient amounts of water helps the body to flush out toxins and to hydrate. Additionally, water is essential to carry nutrients to the body's cells and keep cells hydrated so they function properly. Healthy, well functioning cells contribute to beautiful skin. Proper hydration can also help eliminate the appearance of sunken eyes and dark circles under the eyes. Drinking enough water is one of the most important ways to ensure beautiful skin. How much is enough? Take your weight, divide it by two and drink that many ounces of water per day. If you weigh 150 pounds, drink 75 ounces of water daily. (*Note: Check with a healthcare practitioner before increasing your water intake, particularly if you have kidney issues.*)

Don't Become a "Prune." Prunes are healthy to eat, but you don't want to look like one! Nobody wants wrinkled skin. It is very important to have good fat in your daily diet or you may become a "prune!" While fat sometimes gets a bad reputation, I can tell when people have completely given up eating good fats and oils because their skin sags and develops wrinkles. Additionally, fatty acids are important to the health of cell membranes, which provide a barrier against harmful toxins. Fatty acids help keep cell membranes flexible and permeable to allow nutrients to enter into cells and waste materials to get out. Healthy cell membranes hold more water, which means moister, softer skin.

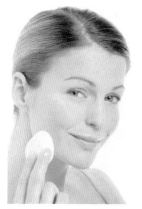

Promote beautiful skin from the inside out!

Omega-3 supplements and beautiful skin go hand in hand. Consuming sufficient amounts of omega-3s can help combat skin dryness—dry skin is one of the symptoms of a fatty acid deficiency. Omega-3s also have anti-inflammatory properties. Inflammation contributes to aging and affects how healthy skin looks and feels.

Individuals suffering from skin disorders may also benefit from omega-3 supplementation. A 2011 study published in *Clinical, Cosmetic and Investigational Dermatology* found that omega-3 supplementation improved severity of symptoms in individuals with mild to moderate psoriasis, an autoimmune disease that causes the skin to develop scaly red and white patches. Omega-3s may also help relieve eczema (itchy, dry skin caused by skin inflammation) and acne.

Depending on your preference, good omega-3s for beautiful skin include **krill oil** and **fish oils** such as salmon oil or calamari oil. In addition to omega-3 fatty acids, krill oil also contains vitamin E and two powerful antioxidants, astaxanthin and canthaxanthin. Krill oil can help fight inflammation and protect the skin from ultraviolet rays from the sun. The omega-3s found in salmon oil and calamari oil can decrease clogged pores, reduces dryness and related problems and improve skin elasticity.

Another category of beneficial fatty acids is gamma linolenic acid (GLA), which is classified as an anti-inflammatory omega-6 fatty acid. My favorite sources of GLA are **borage oil** and **evening primrose oil**.

Neutralize Free Radicals With Resveratrol. Every day, the body replaces damaged cells with new, healthier ones. As we age, this process does not happen as readily. One nutrient that can help support the body in replacing damaged skin cells is resveratrol, a powerful antioxidant phytochemical found abundantly in grape skins and

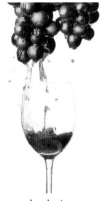

Grapes and red wine may help fight aging by supplying resveratrol.

red wine as well as in blueberries, raspberries, cranberries, peanuts and pistachios. Resveratrol can help the body replace damaged cells more rapidly, slowing the effects of aging.

Oxidation is one of the major causes of skin aging. As a powerful antioxidant, resveratrol can protect the skin from damage due to free radicals, slowing the aging process. A 2010 study published in *PLoS One*, a peer-reviewed journal from the Public Library of Science, reported that resveratrol can protect skin cells against the toxic effect of nitric oxide, a chemical associated with many age-related skin disorders. Researchers concluded that supplementing the diet with resveratrol may help delay or prevent normal skin aging.

Another major cause of skin aging is exposure to ultraviolet (UV) rays from the sun. According to the U.S. Environmental Protection Agency (EPA), "up to *90 percent* of the visible skin changes commonly attributed to aging are caused by the sun. With proper protection from UV radiation, most premature aging of the skin can be avoided." While sunscreen and other measures are vital to protect your skin from the sun's rays, a 2011 study published in *Archives of Biochemistry and Biophysics* reports that taking resveratrol orally can protect the skin against the oxidative stress caused by sun exposure.

Hyaluronic Acid. Another nutrient important for skin health is hyaluronic acid, which occurs naturally in the body. Hyaluronic acid makes up a large part of the skin, helping to repair tissues and functioning as a natural moisturizer. Taken orally, hyaluronic acid can slow skin degradation. Taking hyaluronic acid orally can also help minimize joint pain associated with arthritis. See page 55 for information about using hyaluronic acid topically.

Silica Drops. Silica is a trace element necessary for the formation of *collagen*, a protein that connects and supports the body's tissues, including the skin. Silica is often overlooked as a cosmetic nutrient, but it is one of the most important supplements for healthy skin, beautiful hair, strong bones and hard nails. Sufficient silica in the tissues helps the skin stay flexible and elastic. When skin loses its elasticity, it begins to show signs of aging, such as wrinkles and sagging. Silica can also improve skin tone by helping the body eliminate toxins.

Silica can come from many sources, but my favorite is silica drops from bamboo. Bamboo contains more silica than any other plant source—it contains over 70 percent silica. Other sources of silica include foods that grow underground (such as potatoes, peanuts and beets), wheat bran, soybeans, leafy vegetables (such as spinach, mustard greens, lettuce and cabbage) and brown rice.

Eat Some (Healthy) Fat. Healthy skin needs foods with fats! If you are not getting enough healthy fatty acids in your diet, it shows in your skin. Healthy fats are the building blocks of healthy skin cell membranes. When present in adequate amounts, healthy fats build the skin's natural oil barrier, which keeps the skin hydrated and looking young. Without enough healthy fats, skin can become dry, inflamed and prone to breakouts.

One of my favorite food sources of healthy fats is avocados. Not only do avocados contain healthy monounsaturated fats that help maintain skin integrity, but they are also a good source of other vitamins and minerals important to healthy skin. Avocados contain copper, which helps with skin elasticity and also helps defend against free radicals. Avocados also contain other antioxidants, including vitamins A, D and E and iron.

Along with healthy fats, sufficient protein in the diet is very important for healthy skin. After water, protein is the most common ingredient in skin cells. The body uses protein to replace worn-out skin cells. Protein is made up of amino acids. Amino acids help the body produce collagen, which helps the skin be elastic. Sufficient collagen promotes thicker, healthier skin. The United States Department of Agriculture (USDA) recommends that adult women consume about 46 grams of protein daily and adult men consume about 56 grams.

Outside In

The ingredients you use topically are just as important as the ones you ingest. If you would not eat something, don't put it on your skin! The body absorbs about 60 percent of the substances put on the skin.

The first step in taking care of your skin from the outside in is using the right skincare ingredients. When buying products for topical use, the most important thing is to find products with NO parabens, NO petroleum, NO dyes and NO perfumes. Parabens and petroleum are dangerous xenoestrogens, synthetic dyes are suspected carcinogens and synthetic perfumes are packed full of potentially dangerous chemicals. Protect your skin from the environment—do not expose your skin and body to additional toxins! Throw out any products that contain these harmful ingredients.

The next step is to cleanse your face *every night* using natural products. Products that don't have preservatives and artificial colors in them are more readily found at health food stores than at pharmacies. I suggest cycling through different natural cleansers, since when you continually use the same products, the body gets used to the ingredients and they may not be as effective. I enjoy buying different brands with different ingredients, just as long as they are natural.

Beautiful skin also needs moisturizer. One of the best moisturizers for beautiful skin is hyaluronic acid. We talked about this nutrient in the section about nutrients you should ingest, but hyaluronic acid is also good to apply topically. Hyaluronic acid is the moisture or fluid that supports collagen. Collagen helps keep the skin supple, flexible and resilient. Production of collagen decreases with age, which leads to developing wrinkles. By supporting collagen, hyaluronic acid helps your skin look younger.

Other important topical ingredients for beautiful skin include retinol creams, which help slough off skin to reveal new younger skin, antioxidant creams, vitamin C and alpha lipoic acid.

Another good option for skin care is coconut oil. We will discuss the many health benefits of consuming coconut oil on page 77, but coconut oil is extremely beneficial when applied topically to the skin. Coconut oil is an excellent moisturizer for all skin types and can help prevent skin dryness and flaking. It can also help prevent wrinkles and skin sagging.

With the help of healthy eating and a few nutritional supplements, you can maintain healthy, beautiful skin as you age. Knowing that you look good can also help you feel good!

Mirror Mirror on the Wall . . .
A Daily Skin Routine To Be the Fairest of Them All.

- always cleanse your face before bedtime
- drink plenty of water
- eat good fats
- take nutrients that help repair cells
- use moisturizers during the day and before bedtime
- get sufficient sleep (adults need 7–9 hours per night)

Fight The Fat

Many women gain weight as they enter perimenopause and menopause. Such weight gain may be due to hormonal, genetic and lifestyle factors. But as with many things, just because everyone's doing something does not mean that you should! Weight gain increases the risk of heart disease, stroke, diabetes and breast cancer.

Gaining weight is not inevitable. A few lifestyle changes can help you reverse the weight gain trend. While such changes are not always easy, they are certainly worth it. You will feel better and be healthier in the long term. The pain or discomfort of it will certainly be worth the joy.

Calorie Restriction

Simply stated, to lose weight, you need to burn more calories than you consume. One important way to accomplish this is through calorie restriction. Calorie restriction does not mean starving, it simply means eating fewer calories.

Calorie restriction can have many benefits in addition to weight loss. For one thing, calorie restriction can fight aging. Groups that research ways to encourage longevity, such as the National Institute on Aging and Life Extension®, suggest different advice, but the majority agree that calorie restriction slows the aging process. Calorie restriction can turn on your longevity genes and turn back the clock of aging.

Calorie restriction helps fight aging because it places less demand on the organs of the body. You require a lot from your body each day. All the organs in the body are constantly working to process and detoxify the things you take into your body. The lungs, intestines and pancreas work and work and work, and over time, they can "run out of steam." Eating less can help prevent negative effects in the body because the body has less to process.

The idea that calorie restriction increases longevity dates to 1935. Dr. Clive M. McCay Ph. D., a nutritionist at Cornell University, found that a 30 percent decrease in caloric intake in mice led to a 40 percent increase in lifespan. In recent years, scientists have found that calorie restriction leads to similar lifespan increases in other animals. While human studies are still preliminary, a 2009 article in *Current Opinion in Gastroenterology* reported that "calorie restriction with adequate nutrition protects against obesity, type 2 diabetes, hypertension and atherosclerosis."

The key to calorie restriction is consuming the nutrients that the body needs while cutting calorie intake by 20–30 percent. For an individual following a 2,000 calorie/day diet, calorie restriction would mean cutting back to 1,400–1,600 calories/day. Calorie restriction requires careful planning to ensure adequate nutrition. Consult a healthcare practitioner before beginning a calorie restricted diet.

Eliminate Wheat and Gluten

Gluten is a protein composite found in grains of barley, rye, wheat and wheat relatives. It is found in most breads, pastas and many other food products that contain wheat flour. Wheat and gluten are very common allergies. According to the Celiac Disease Foundation, one in 133 adults are gluten or wheat sensitive. Many people don't realize that their runny noses, coughs, earaches and skin rashes may be caused by wheat and gluten in their diets.

I often meet people who complain that no matter how much they exercise or cut calories, they still cannot lose weight. I have found that often when these same people give up wheat and gluten, weight loss follows. Often, after eliminating wheat and gluten, the body starts metabolizing fat more quickly. Bloating and weight gain are common in people with a gluten intolerance. Eliminating wheat and gluten can lead to less bloating and flatter abs. For those individuals, when eating a gluten-free diet, the bloat in the stomach goes away and they have more energy.

Many wheat and gluten-free breads and other products are now available. Gluten-free wheat alternatives include rice, corn, buckwheat, millet and quinoa. Gluten-free flours include almond, chestnut, sorghum, amaranth, rice and corn. Different grains have different tastes and textures and usually cannot be substituted 1:1 with flour, but do a little research before diving into gluten-free cooking and baking. Gluten-free cookbooks, cake mixes, helpful blogs and websites are abundant. After a bit of research a whole new world of fabulous grains, nuts and seeds will open up and bring on a healthier lifestyle.

Balance Your Blood Sugar

Being overweight or obese can contribute to many degenerative diseases, including diabetes. Diabetes is a disease where the body has trouble regulating blood sugar (glucose) levels due to a problem with insulin, a hormone produced in the pancreas. Insulin allows glucose, the body's main source of energy, to enter into cells to be used as energy or stored as fat. Without insulin, the cells are deprived access to glucose and sugars build up in the blood. Being overweight or obese can contribute to insulin resistance, a related condition where cells become resistant to insulin and less effective at controlling blood sugar.

The two main forms of diabetes are type 1 diabetes and type 2 diabetes. Type 1 diabetes occurs when the body does

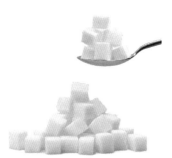

not produce sufficient insulin. Type 2 diabetes occurs when insulin is no longer effective in the body. Type 2 diabetes was once referred to as "adult-onset diabetes." However, it is now commonly diagnosed in children as well as adults. The primary risk factors

Blood sugar imbalances can lead to degenerative diseases like diabetes.

for type 2 diabetes include family history of diabetes, aging and obesity. Statistics say that more than 85 percent of people with type 2 diabetes are overweight. In some cases, individuals with type 2 diabetes can normalize their blood sugar levels through diet and exercise.

Many researchers blame the increase in children with type 2 diabetes on the corresponding rise in childhood obesity. A 2006 study published in the *Journal of the American Medical Association* found that obesity in children ages 6 to 19 tripled between 1980 and 2002 and continued to rise between 2002 and 2006.

Obesity and diabetes are closely linked. A study co-sponsored by the CDC and the National Institute of Diabetes and Digestive and Kidney Diseases (NIDDK) called SEARCH found that 30 percent of children with diabetes could be classified as overweight, while 44 percent were at risk of becoming overweight.

These alarming statistics have a lot to do with the fact that sugar is found in many processed foods. Eating simple, refined sugars causes sharp rises in blood sugar. In response, the body signals the pancreas to release insulin to process the sugar in the blood. In a person with type 2 diabetes, typically the body has become resistant to insulin and does not respond to insulin the way it normally would. Sugar accumulates in the blood, which can lead to fatigue, slow wound healing and problems with eyes and vision.

However, healthcare practitioners suggest that diabetes is preventable in six out of 10 cases. What can you do? Diet can be a contributing factor in developing diabetes. Two main contributors to both obesity and diabetes are consumption of white flour and sugar. Such refined carbohydrates provide little nutritional value while wreaking havoc on blood sugar levels. An excess amount of white flour and white sugar in the diet can increase the risk of developing various diseases, including heart disease and diabetes.

White flour and sugar also stimulate the appetite and may cause cravings. Breads, pastas, desserts and sweetened drinks load nutritionally-empty calories into one's diet. Eliminating white flour and sugar can help reduce caloric intake, which encourages weight loss. And replacing white flour and sugar with whole grains and natural sweeteners can also improve the overall nutritional quality of the diet. Whole grains contain more fiber, which take longer to digest and release glucose more slowly. Slower glucose release helps maintain blood sugar balance.

Often, food choices are motivated more by emotions than hunger. Don't fall into this trap! Pay attention to your emotions and don't allow how you feel to trigger what and when you eat.

Two nutrients that may be particularly helpful for balancing blood sugar are the mineral chromium and biotin (vitamin B_7). In a 2008 study in *Diabetes/ Metabolism Research and Reviews*, researchers looked at 447 individuals with poorly controlled diabetes. Half received 600 mcg of chromium with 2 mg of biotin, while the other half received a placebo. Both blood sugar control and fasting blood glucose levels improved in those who received the chromium/biotin supplement.

Biotin may also play a role in helping prevent *diabetic neuropathy*, which is characterized by numbness and tingling in the hands and feet and is associated with poor glucose control. About 60–70 percent of individuals with diabetes suffer from mild neuropathy.

Good Food in All the Right Places

The key to losing weight and becoming more healthy is to go "back to basics" with food. The "food" that ads try to get us to eat is often not really food at all—it is chemicals and genetically modified organisms (GMOs) with preservatives, artificial color, sugar and sodium.

In GMOs, the food's original DNA structure has been changed. Scientists genetically modify plants for many reasons—to make them resistant to herbicides, or to increase their shelf life. However, scientists are still unsure how the body metabolizes GMOs. Some evidence suggests that modifying the genetic code of foods can alter the immune system, increase inflammation and increase the number of allergic reactions to foods. In other words, the body may not recognize a GMO as "real" food.

Don't be a scientific experiment! Start looking for food in all the right places. Plan your diet around fruits and vegetables, NOT processed food from a box or can. And if you are someone who claims to not like vegetables, try a fresh organic vegetable. It's delicious! Go back to basics. It will make a huge difference in how you feel!

Get Moving!

Exercise must be part of any wellness program. The importance of exercise cannot be overlooked in the quest to extend life while reducing the chances of developing debilitating diseases. The body is jointed, which means it is meant to move! In case you are not sure some of good reasons to exercise, here are a few: Exercise can help make weight management much easier. It has an almost immediate effect for helping moods and managing stress. Exercise can lower blood pressure, help diabetes and improve digestion. Exercise helps with blood circulation, which can improve memory and heart function. Exercise makes the body physically stronger and can help prevent and even reverse osteoporosis.

Include resistance training (some kind of exercise using weights) in your exercise program because it helps strengthen bones. Many people take calcium supplements to fight osteoporosis, but in order for the body to absorb calcium and other minerals, there must be a demand for these minerals in the bones. Bones need to be compressed and pulled in order for the body to realize it needs to absorb minerals from the foods we eat and the mineral vitamins we take. Resistance exercises help create that demand.

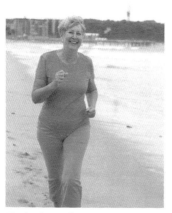

Find a form of exercise you enjoy and get moving!

A caveat to exercise: do not make yourself miserable by forcing yourself to exercise in ways you don't enjoy. It helps to be creative. Every little bit you do counts. Turn some music on and dance while you clean your house!

Other Weight Control Tips:

- drink more water—half your body weight in ounces (as suggested on page 50)
- don't skip meals
- eat protein with each meal (protein boosts metabolism and helps the body burn fat)
- consume more fiber
- eat your large meal of the day before 5 p.m.

Do Not Waste Energy

A discussion of health and balance would not be complete without discussing digestion. The gastrointestinal (GI) system is very complex. Its role is to extract nutrients and water from the food and liquid ingested, and prepare such nutrients so that the body can use them for nourishment. For digestion to work properly, the GI system needs to break down fats, carbohydrates and protein so they can enter the bloodstream. Such breakdown is accomplished by digestive enzymes working in harmony with each other. If any part of this system does not fulfill its role, symptoms such as heartburn, acid reflux, bloating, gas, pain, constipation or loose bowel movements can result. Ultimately, if nutrients are not absorbed, we cannot survive.

Digestion is also important for energy. Each person has a certain amount of energy available to them—their "100 percent." Everyone's 100 percent is different. Your 100 percent might be more or less than mine. But all you have is your 100 percent, no more. And how you use that 100 percent is the difference in feeling happy or exhausted, stressed and anxious.

Digestion is one area in which energy is easily wasted. Breaking food into particles that the digestive tract can absorb requires quite a bit of ATP energy. From the muscular action of chewing to the involuntary muscle movements that push food through the intestines, digestion can be an energy-sapping process. If you eat a heavy, fat-laden meal, you can use up to 60 percent of all your available energy to digest it. And if you are using 60 percent of your energy to digest food, that leaves only 40 percent of your energy for work, family or personal time.

Your energy is a valuable and finite resource. Most of us lead stressful lives, with constant demands. Many of us give and give and give . . . and that requires a lot of energy. So don't waste your precious energy on digestion!

A few factors can affect the amount of energy we need for digestion. Difficulties with digestion are often caused by the amount of food consumed. Everybody's stomach has a limit. When you overeat, the digestive system can be overwhelmed by the amount of food that it needs to process. Chronic overeating can severely overtax the digestive system, draining energy.

Instead of eating until you are "stuffed" or beyond full, watch your portions and leave the table when you are almost full. Try adopting the Japanese custom of *hara hachi bunme*—which means you stop eating when you feel 80 percent full. Following this practice requires being aware of when you are hungry and can help you avoid mindless eating. Eating a little less with every meal can mean spending a little less energy on digestion, leaving you a little more of your "100 percent."

The Okinawa diet, based on eating habits of people who live on the Japanese islands of Ryukyu, offers an excellent example. Okinawans have the longest life expectancy of any people in the world—roughly 29 percent of Okinawans live to be 100 years old, about four times more than in Western countries. Researchers credit the traditional Okinawan diet for their longevity.

The Okinawa diet is centered on lean animal proteins and plant proteins, particularly from yellow and green vegetables. Those following the Okinawa diet eat no red meat, eggs or dairy, which can be hard for the body to digest. The principle of *hara hachi bunme* is also central to the Okinawa diet.

Slow Food

Related to how much you eat is how fast you eat. When your stomach and intestines are empty and your blood sugar levels are low, your stomach sends signals to your brain that relays the sensation of hunger. The same thing happens in reverse when you eat and your stomach becomes full—the stomach signals the brain that it has enough food. However, this signal is not instantaneous. If you eat too quickly, you can stuff yourself before the stomach has a chance to signal your brain that it has had enough. Avoid this predicament by relaxing, eating slowly and enjoying your food!

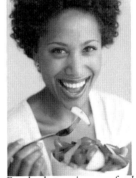

Eat slowly to enjoy your food and fight weight gain.

In a study published in the *Journal of the American Dietetic Association* in 2008, researchers studied the caloric intake of 30 healthy women for two meals. For both meals, the women were given a large plate of pasta and told to eat as much as they wanted. However, for the first meal, they were told to eat quickly, while for the second meal, they were told to eat slowly and chew each bite 20 times. In the first meal, the women consumed an average of 646 calories before they felt full, while in the second meal, they consumed an average of 579 calories before feeling full. Not only did the women consume fewer calories, but they also reported feeling full an hour after the meal. The researchers concluded that "eating slowly may help to maximize satiation and reduce energy intake within meals."

JUST SAY "NO."

The kinds of foods you eat can also have a big impact on the digestive process. Certain types of foods are more difficult to process. While healthy fats are essential to good health, fats are also the most difficult type of food for the body to digest. The body particularly struggles to digest *hydrogenated* fats and *trans* fats—types of fat generally not found in nature.

Hydrogenated fats are solid fats, created by adding hydrogen molecules to liquid oils. Examples of hydrogenated fats include margarine, shortening and prepared foods such as pastries, breads, cake mixes, pie crusts, whipped toppings and some frozen breakfast foods such as waffles. Hydrogen is even sometimes added to peanut butter, to help prolong its shelf life.

Adding hydrogen means that the fat's carbon bonds do not separate, which extends the fat's shelf life. However, the added hydrogen also makes it difficult for the body to separate carbon bonds and absorb the fat, making it more difficult for the body to digest. Additionally, hydrogenated fats convert to trans fats when heated. Trans fats have been linked to increased risk of heart disease and cancer.

Two other types of fats are saturated and unsaturated fats. Saturated fats are found in dairy and meat products as well as certain plant oils, such as coconut oil, cocoa butter and palm oils. They are solid at room temperature. While animal fats raise blood cholesterol levels because they contain cholesterol, saturated fats from plants contain *phytosterols* instead, which do not raise cholesterol.

Unsaturated fats from vegetable oils are liquid at room temperature, but because they are unsaturated, they oxidize quickly, so they contribute to free radical damage in the body when consumed.

Furthermore, unsaturated vegetable oils such as safflower, corn, cottonseed and soybean oils contain a prevalence of omega-6 fatty acids. Many Western diets contain so many omega-6 fatty acids that they are out of balance with omega-3 fatty acids. This imbalance has created inflammatory conditions that are partially responsible for the chronic inflammation that lead to many Western diseases. Generally, naturally occurring saturated fats, such as butter or coconut oil, are better alternatives in cooking than unsaturated vegetable oils or hydrogenated margarine or shortening.

To make digestion easier and avoid draining your energy unnecessarily, avoid hydrogenated and trans fats completely! When cooking, use healthy saturated fats instead of hydrogenated vegetable oils. While saturated fats are generally viewed negatively, there are some exceptions. Coconut oil is a particularly healthy choice for cooking and baking. (See page 77 for information about the health benefits of coconut oil.)

In addition to changing fat choices, certain types of food can encourage more efficient digestion. As previously mentioned, include whole grains (found in whole wheat bread, oatmeal, brown rice and more) and sufficient amounts of fiber in your diet. According to the USDA, adults should consume 14 grams of fiber per 1,000 calories consumed.

Such measures can help ensure that the digestive system can digest food without wasting energy. Providing the body with the right kinds of foods, including healthy fats, also ensures that the body has a sufficient supply of the nutrients needed. The more energy you can conserve through proper digestion, the more energy you have to do the things you need and want to do.

Supplement Healthy Digestion

No matter what you eat, if it is not broken down properly in the body, the nutrients from the food cannot be absorbed. In order to absorb nutrients from food, the body breaks down complex foods into soluble substances. Digestive enzymes are proteins that the body uses to break down food; hence, another important factor in efficient digestion is the body's supply of digestive enzymes.

Glands in the mouth, stomach, pancreas and small intestines secrete digestive enzymes. Raw foods also contain enzymes that the body can use to help with digestion. So we shouldn't have any problem getting all the digestive enzymes we need, right?

Unfortunately, many people do not get as many digestive enzymes as they need. Why? Cooking foods at temperatures above 118 degrees Fahrenheit destroys any enzymes the food contains. Since most of the foods we eat are cooked and processed, we often consume foods that are devoid of enzymes. And with age, the body produces fewer digestive enzymes.

If the body does not have sufficient digestive enzymes to break down the food one consumes, food is often stored as fat. Digestive enzyme supplements can be the answer to digestion woes. Different types of digestive enzymes can be helpful for different situations.

General Digestive Enzymes. The first important type of digestive enzyme is a general digestive enzyme. This type of digestive enzyme can break up fats, carbohydrates and proteins. Specific types of general digestive enzymes include *protease*, which helps digest protein.

Good sources of protease include bromelain, which is derived from pineapple stem, and papain, derived from the stem and sap of papaya. Other general digestive enzymes include *amylase*, which helps digest carbohydrates and starch, and *lipase*, which helps digest fat. Look for a digestive enzyme supplement that supplies different types of digestive enzymes to digest different types of foods.

Pancreatic Enzymes. Pancreatin is a type of pancreatic enzyme generally made from enzymes from pig or cow pancreas. Pancreatin contains enzymes that help break down proteins, fats and carbohydrates. Because such enzymes can be destroyed by stomach acid, take them 20 minutes before eating so they will pass quickly into the upper digestive system where they work as general digestive enzymes.

Pancreatin contains protease, lipase and amylase, as well as *trypsin*, a type of protease that helps break down protein so the body can digest it. Pancreatin is useful when the pancreas does not supply the digestive system with enough enzymes for proper digestion.

One other interesting benefit of pancreatic enzymes is to prevent hangovers! Hangovers happen in part because alcohol decreases the body's secretion of enzymes, inhibiting the body's ability to break down nutrients. As a result, excess alcohol circulates in the blood, causing stress to the body. Pancreatic enzymes help consume undigested protein in the blood, cleansing the blood and preventing hangovers (for some people). To use pancreatic enzymes for this purpose, try taking four 500 mg capsules or tablets before drinking alcohol.

Hydrochloric Acid (HCl). Hydrochloric acid is a main component of gastric acid, which is secreted in the stomach. Hydrochloric acid has two important functions: it helps prevent infection by destroying harmful organisms and it plays an important role in digesting food. The body's production of HCl tends to decrease with age, which can lead to problems digesting food. Supplementing the diet with HCl can help the digestive system function optimally.

As previously mentioned, HCl is also necessary for the body to break apart mineral salts (such as calcium carbonate, magnesium citrate and other "–ates"). If you do not have enough acid in your intestines, your body will not be able to absorb calcium or other minerals from food or supplements.

Many people think that they have enough acid in their stomachs because they experience acid reflux, or heartburn. Acid reflux symptoms may actually mean that the stomach does not have enough acid or that there is a hiatal hernia that causes acid to spray up into the esophagus. Check with a healthcare practitioner, as chronic acid reflux can lead to serious complications, including esophageal cancer.

If you experience indigestion caused by too little stomach acid but do not have reflux or heartburn, an HCl supplement can aid digestion. Look for HCl with *pepsin*, a digestive enzyme produced by the stomach that helps digest protein. The stomach needs HCl to produce pepsin, so individuals with insufficient stomach acid often lack pepsin as well.

Supporting digestive health can also help you avoid illnesses that drain energy. Since over 70 percent of the immune system is housed in the gut, healthy digestion plays a very important part in immune system function.

Clean Up Your Act

According to the World Health Organization (WHO), 24 percent of the disease burden worldwide is due to environmental factors, such as exposure to toxins. The

EPA confirms that most people are exposed to thousands of chemicals every day from food, water and the environment. Subtle, long-term exposure to toxins can cause toxins to accumulate throughout the entire body.

The body's natural detoxification system, (the lungs, liver, kidneys, gastrointestinal tract and skin) does a great job. But when the body is exposed to massive amounts of environmental pollutants, the body's natural detoxification system can become overwhelmed. The body may need a little help to deal with so many toxins.

Internal cleansing is also very important. The question is not *if* you should cleanse but *how often*. I suggest cleansing three to four times a year to help with weight, energy, skin health, elimination and digestion. Use a general, gentle two-week cleanse (not a "drastic" cleanse that can sometimes do more harm than good). Look for products that gently cleanse the whole body and help with toxin and waste elimination.

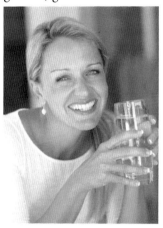

Drinking pure filtered water is a crucial part of cleansing the body.

While using a body cleansing supplementary kit, drink at least 64 ounces of water daily. Limit or eliminate consumption of foods containing sugar, wheat, gluten and dairy. Such foods tend to slow down the cleansing process.

For one day of your cleanse, try my "detox" soup. Eat the soup with the vegetables throughout the day, and drink at least 64 ounces of pure, filtered water. After drinking just the soup for one day, your skin will glow and you will have more energy.

DETOX SOUP RECIPE

Ingredients:

- 1 qt organic vegetable broth OR organic chicken broth
- 1 qt pure, filtered water
- 2 large onions, sliced or diced
- 1 bulb of garlic, peeled and separated into cloves
- 2 beets, cut into cubes
- 4 stalks of celery, cut into 2-inch pieces
- 4 carrots, cut into bite-size pieces
- 2 parsnips, cut into bite-size pieces
- 2 cups kale
- 2 cups spinach
- 1 tsp black pepper
- 2 tablespoons paprika
- 1 tsp cayenne pepper (if you like a spicy soup)

Directions:

In an 8-quart pot, add 1 quart of organic vegetable broth or organic chicken broth. Add 1 quart of pure, filtered water. Add vegetables and spices and bring to a boil, stirring occasionally. Simmer for 15 or 20 minutes or until vegetables reach the texture you desire.

Note: If you have diabetes or are hypoglycemic, do not fast. For such healthcare conditions only use this soup in addition to a regular, healthful diet.

Your Fountain of Youth

Going Coconuts

Coconut oil is one of the healthiest and most beneficial types of oils. But if you check the nutrition facts box on the label, you might find that statement hard to believe. Many people are afraid of fat, especially saturated fat, and coconut oil is full of saturated fat. But we need fat! Don't be afraid of fat. When you eat *good* fats (found naturally in foods like avocados, coconuts, flaxseeds, olives and fish), the body feels satiated for longer periods of time.

The saturated fats in coconut oil mostly come from a medium-chain fatty acid called *lauric acid*. The body converts lauric acid to monolaurin, which has antiviral, antibacterial and antifungal properties. Monolaurin can help fight disease-causing bacteria, including *Listeria monocytogenes* (the leading cause of food poisoning deaths in the United States) and *Helicobacter pylori* (a bacteria associated with the development of stomach ulcers).

Unlike the long-chain fatty acids found in red meats, full-fat dairy products and foods fried in vegetable oil, the body can easily absorb medium-chain fatty acids. Medium-chain fatty acids like lauric acid help the body burn excess calories, which means that consuming coconut oil may help with weight loss. Getting enough fat in the diet can help you eat less and feel more satisfied, because fats naturally suppress appetite by slowing the emptying of the stomach.

As a medium-chain fatty acid, coconut oil is particularly helpful. The body processes medium-chain fatty acids differently from other fats. Instead of being stored in the body as fat, the body immediately uses medium-chain fatty acids to create energy.

Coconut oil has many other health benefits. A study published in 2009 in *Lipids* found that coconut oil may help combat high blood cholesterol. The study compared levels of HDL ("good" cholesterol) and LDL ("bad" cholesterol) in two groups of obese women. (Higher HDL and lower LDL levels are associated with a decreased risk of heart disease.) The researchers found that the group that took a nutritional supplement of 30 mL of coconut oil each day experienced higher HDL levels and lower LDL levels.

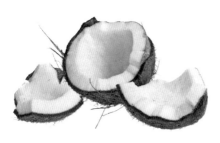

Coconut oil is one of the most healthful cooking oils.

Coconut oil is ideal for cooking. Most oils, even those that are considered "healthy," can become dangerous when they are heated. When heat is introduced to many oils (whether they begin in liquid or solid form), they become oxidized and can become carcinogenic. Coconut oil does not oxidize at high temperatures, making it a safe and delicious alternative to other oils.

Coconut oil also does not need to be refrigerated. In cold weather, it will become solid, and in warm weather it will become a liquid, but coconut oil is safe to use whether in liquid or solid form.

Coconut oil is only healthy in its natural form. Some coconut oil manufacturers process coconut oil in a way that removes its beneficial lauric acid, transforming coconut oil into another dangerous, artery-clogging fat. Avoid refined hydrogenated coconut oil and use only virgin and organic forms.

As an added bonus, coconut oil also provides great natural nutrition for hair! Massage coconut oil directly into your scalp to keep your hair free of dandruff and lice and to nourish damaged hair, or look for hair care products that contain organic, virgin coconut oil as an ingredient.

B Positive

B-complex vitamins are important for all aspects of the body, especially for women. Vitamin B-complex is a family made up of eight vitamins—B_1 (thiamine), B_2 (riboflavin), B_3 (niacin), B_5 (pantothenic acid), B_6 (pyridoxine), B_7 (biotin), B_9 (folic acid) and B_{12} (cyanocobalamin, methycobalamin and other cobalamins). Each of the B-complex vitamins is important for optimal function of the body.

The B-complex vitamins play many important roles in the body. They primarily are involved in energy release and in certain blood functions. They help the body metabolize proteins, fats and carbohydrates. They help build cells and deliver nutrients to cells. Some B-complex vitamins, particularly folic acid, help lower the risk of birth defects such as spina bifida, while biotin supports healthy hair, nails and skin. B-complex vitamins, particularly B_6, B_9 and B_{12}, are necessary to break down *homocysteine*, an amino acid associated with increased risk of heart disease.

Everyone has some homocysteine in the blood, and normally it does not cause any problems. The body produces homocysteine from methionine, an amino acid found in meats, seafood, dairy products and eggs. B-complex vitamins, especially B_6, B_9 and B_{12}, use homocysteine to produce other compounds, including glutathione, a powerful antioxidant. However, without adequate supplies of B-complex vitamins, homocysteine can build up in the body. Elevated homocysteine levels are associated with atherosclerosis, or thickening of artery walls. A 2002 study published in the *Journal of the American Medical Association* reported that supplementing the diet with vitamins B_9 and B_{12} helped lower levels of homocysteine in the body.

Vitamin B-complex has many positive effects on the body. The B-vitamins are good for anti-aging, energy, anxiety and mood and hormonal imbalances. B-vitamins can help fight heart disease and stroke. Vitamin B-complex is very helpful for fighting the harmful effects stress can have on the body.

ANTI-AGING

The B-vitamin family may help fight a variety of effects of aging, including memory loss, reduced cognitive performance and problems with eyesight. The body uses vitamin B_1 to produce neurotransmitters that are important for memory and mental performance. A deficiency of vitamin B_6 is associated with Alzheimer's disease. And a study published in 2005 in the *American Journal of Clinical Nutrition* found that high homocysteine levels and low levels of B-vitamins correlated with cognitive impairment in aging men.

The B-vitamins can also help maintain eyesight by fighting cataracts, a clouding on the lens of the eye caused by free radical damage to proteins in the eye. As the lens of the eye becomes clouded, it can become unable to focus and properly admit light. Cataracts can lead to a gradual, painless loss of vision. According to the WHO, age-related cataracts cause 48 percent of blindness cases worldwide. The B-vitamins can fight the protein deterioration that leads to cataracts by helping protect glutathione in the eye. A deficiency of riboflavin has been linked with developing cataracts.

ENERGY

Many of the B-vitamins are extremely important to energy production. A thiamine deficiency results in beriberi, a disease characterized by extreme weakness and fatigue, and niacin helps enzymes convert nutrients into energy.

Perhaps most significantly, riboflavin plays a vital role in the production of ATP, the source of energy for the body's cells. Any time a muscle moves, ATP provides the energy needed to produce movement. Hence, insufficient riboflavin stores interfere with ATP production, which can cause energy reserves to become depleted. Without riboflavin to help create ATP, the body can become lethargic and sluggish.

Anxiety and Mood

The powerful effect of B-vitamins on mood is partly due to the role of B-vitamins in preventing damage to the nervous system. Vitamin B_{12} plays a particularly important role in maintaining myelin, the fatty sheath that surrounds nerves, protecting nerves and promoting their growth.

A deficiency in any of the B-complex vitamins can lead to mood swings, unstable moods and depression. Information on how the brain and moods work is unclear, but the body may use vitamin B-complex to create serotonin, which is an important neurotransmitter that can contribute to stable moods.

Hormonal Imbalances

As many as three in four women suffer from premenstrual syndrome (PMS). PMS is characterized by a group of symptoms that usually begin one to two weeks before menstruation and typically end when menstruation begins. Symptoms include bloating and weight gain, irritability, breast tenderness or pain, headaches and joint pain.

Hormonal changes often trigger PMS symptoms, but researchers have also linked PMS to low levels of certain vitamins and minerals. For many years, nutritionists have recommended B-vitamin supplements to women suffering from PMS. In a study published in 2011 in the *American Journal of Clinical Nutrition*, researchers spent 10 years studying 3,025 women who did not have PMS symptoms at the beginning of the study. After the 10-year study, researchers reported that women who consumed high quantities of riboflavin had a 35 percent lower risk of developing PMS than women who consumed low quantities. The researchers also reported that consuming large amounts of thiamine also lowered the risk of PMS. Vitamin B_6 can help reduce water retention, a major cause of PMS bloating.

Vitamin B-complex can help with other hormonal balances as well. The B-vitamins play a role in producing all of the body's hormones. Vitamins B_6 and B_{12} can help manage estrogen dominance by helping the liver excrete excess estrogen.

STROKE

According to 2011 data released by the American Heart Association (AHA), strokes cause one out of every 18 deaths in the United States. A stroke happens when a blood clot blocks an artery or blood vessel, interrupting the flow of blood and oxygen to the brain. The brain's cells need oxygen to function, so without oxygen, brain cells begin to die and brain damage can occur. As mentioned, high levels of homocysteine can contribute to atherosclerosis, which in turn contributes to the development of blood clots.

Studies indicate that by helping reduce homocysteine in the blood, B-complex vitamins may also help lower the risk of stroke. A large-scale study published in 2006 in the *New England Journal of Medicine* tracked 5,500 men and women who had been diagnosed with heart disease. Half of the group was given a B-vitamin supplement (containing 2.5 mg folic acid, 50 mg vitamin B_6 and 1 mg vitamin B_{12}). The researchers reported that those who took the supplements were 25 percent less likely to experience strokes.

STRESS

Many health problems are related to stress. Heart disease, digestion problems, depression, anxiety and many other diseases and disorders are at least partially caused by stress. But B-complex vitamins are a great way to help the body fight stress. As mentioned, the B-vitamins can help support mental health and energy and fight depression, all of which help keep the body in better shape to combat stress.

A few of the B-vitamins are particularly helpful. Thiamine can support a healthy nervous system and healthy mental attitude, both of which are important for fighting stress. Vitamin B_6 is required to synthesize serotonin, which helps the body cope with depression, anxiety and stress. Folic acid is also very important. Without adequate folic acid, the body can become depressed and fatigued, which contributes to stress. And vitamin B_5 can help strengthen the immune system so that the body can avoid illness.

All of the B-complex vitamins are water-soluble, meaning they are absorbed directly into the blood and the body eliminates any excess through the urine. Hence, the chance of taking too much vitamin B-complex is low—the body eliminates anything it does not need. It also means that we need to consume B-complex vitamins regularly to replenish the body's supply.

Since all the B-complex vitamins are important, don't take just one! All of the B-vitamins work in tandem, and taking a supplement of just one of the B-complex vitamins can cause an imbalance. I suggest adults take a 50 mg B-complex vitamin two times a day with food. Additionally, I suggest taking vitamin B_{12} as a chewable (vitamin B_{12} is best absorbed sublingually, or through the tissues under the tongue). Vitamin B_{12} is found in B-complex supplements, but supplementing extra B_{12} as a chewable can help ensure the body can absorb it. If desired, add extra supplements of a particular B-vitamin to boost your body's supply.

Queen Bee

Another type of "B" can have many beneficial effects— bee products! Bee pollen, royal jelly, propolis and honey can help increase energy and stamina and have natural antibiotic, anti-inflammatory and anti-aging properties. Royal jelly is one of the best sources of naturally-occurring B-vitamins available. Many B-vitamin supplements are synthetic, so if you are looking for a natural source of B-vitamins, try royal jelly.

(*Note: See a healthcare practitioner before using bee products, particularly if you are allergic to any bee product, including honey and bee venom, or if you are allergic to pollen.*)

Bee Pollen. Bees gather pollen from flowers and flowering trees and mix it with enzymes and nectar to form bee pollen granules. These tiny granules contain small amounts of B-complex vitamins, including B_1, B_2, B_3, B_5, B_6 and B_{12}. Bee pollen also contains small amounts of vitamins A, C, D and E, as well as proteins, minerals and amino acids.

Due to its nutrient content, bee pollen is a great natural energy enhancer. In addition, a 2006 Japanese study on rats published in the *Journal of Health Science* suggested that bee pollen helped stimulate bone growth. However no human studies have been done to date. Bee pollen may help stimulate the growth of bone DNA in humans but more research needs to be done.

Royal Jelly. Royal jelly is a creamy liquid used to nourish bee larvae for their first three days of life and the queen bee throughout her life. It contains all of the B-vitamins and is particularly rich in pantothenic acid, which has potent anti-stress properties.

Like bee pollen, royal jelly is a natural energy booster. It can also help fight symptoms of depression. And royal jelly may also help regulate hormones, helping with symptoms of menopause. A study published in 2004 in *Medscape General Medicine* reported that a dietary supplement containing royal jelly alleviated menopausal symptoms, including hormonal headaches and hot flashes, in a group of menopausal women.

Propolis. Bees make propolis by adding wax to tree resin. In the Greek language, *propolis* means defender of the city. Bees use propolis to defend their hive from infection, by sealing cracks or holes in the hive's structure. Propolis contains vitamins A, C, D and E as well as a mix of minerals, flavonoids and amino acids.

Propolis has antibacterial and antiviral properties. It defends the bees against any outside contaminants or intruders and also sterilizes the bees upon entering the hive. For humans, propolis can be used both as a topical ointment and as a dietary supplement for its antibacterial effects. Propolis is also an excellent natural anti-inflammatory.

Honey. Bees make honey from nectar in flower blossoms combined with their own enzymes. Honey is a natural sweetener that has been used as both food and medicine since ancient times. It contains a variety of nutrients, including calcium and potassium along with trace amounts of vitamin C and B-complex.

Honey, too, is an excellent natural energy booster. The National Honey Board suggests adding honey to water or using it as a sweetener in snacks for a natural energy boost. Honey is a combination of different sugars, such as monosaccharides (fructose and glucose), disaccharides (sucrose and maltose) and oligosaccharides, a more complex sugar. Sugars comprise 95–98 percent of honey.

Research suggests that many of honey's more complex sugars are not found in the flower nectar but are formed during the ripening of the honey in the comb caused by the bee enzymes and the natural acids of the honey.

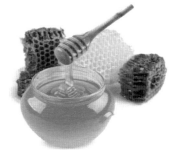

Bee products may boost energy and fight stress, among other benefits.

Raw honey may be especially beneficial. Raw honey is not heated or processed, so it retains vitamins, enzymes, antioxidants and other nutritional components found in honey in its natural state. Raw honey contains beneficial phytonutrients including caffeic acid, methyl caffeate, phenylethyl caffeate and phenylethyl dimethylcaffeate. Such phytonutrients support the immune system and help the body fight colds and flu due to their antibacterial, antiviral and antifungal properties.

Note: Do not feed honey to infants under one year old. Honey can contain Clostridium botulinum *spores that can cause infant botulism, a rare disease that affects the nervous systems of children under one year old.*

Friendly Fats

As we've talked about, fats don't always deserve their bad reputation. The right fats in the right amounts can be extremely beneficial in improving how you present yourself to the world—how you look, how you move and how you feel.

Essential fatty acids, or EFAs, are a form of polyunsaturated fat. They are called "essential" because your body needs them for good health, but is unable to produce them. Essential fatty acids are divided into categories depending on their chemical structures. Two of the main categories include omega-3 and omega-6 fatty acids.

We have already discussed several benefits of omega-3s and omega-6s. Omega-3s and omega-6s come from different sources and have different roles in the body. Generally, omega-6s encourage inflammation while omega-3s discourage it. Inflammation is an important part of the body's immune response, but chronic or prolonged inflammation is associated with aging and disease, including rheumatoid arthritis, heart disease, Alzheimer's disease and depression. Often, diets in the U.S. have an imbalance of omegas—too high in omega-6s and not enough omega-3s.

Beneficial omega-3 fatty acids have three forms: alpha-linolenic acid (an essential fatty acid found in plant oils), EPA (eicosapentaenoic acid) and DHA (docosahexaenoic acid), found in fish, krill and calamari oils. Beneficial omega-6 fatty acids have two forms: linoleic acid and gamma-linolenic acid (GLA). Many people get sufficient omega-6 linoleic acid from their diets, but healthful sources of GLA include borage oil, evening primrose oil and black currant oil. Too much linoleic acid however, can lead to chronic inflammation as it is the precursor to inflammatory eicosanoids.

In addition to skin benefits of omega-3s (discussed on pages 50–51), EFAs have a host of other benefits. Because of their anti-inflammatory and nourishing properties, EFAs can support the health of the heart, joints, brain, eyes and nervous system.

Heart

The American Heart Association (AHA) first described the potential benefits of fish oil in 1996. A report published in 1996 in *Circulation* advised that consuming omega-3s from oily fish such as salmon, herring, mackerel, anchovies and sardines could benefit individuals with coronary heart disease. Since the publication of that report, studies and research trials have established that omega-3s may have many cardiovascular benefits.

In 2003, the AHA released an updated statement about the potential benefits of fish oils, published in *Arteriosclerosis, Thrombosis, and Vascular Biology*. According to the statement, adequate consumption of omega-3 fatty acids decreases the risk of dying from a heart attack and also decreases the risk of suffering a stroke. In the same article, the AHA also reported that regularly consuming oily fish can lower *triglycerides* (a type of fat found in the blood) and blood pressure and decrease the risk of blood clots.

The AHA recommends two to four grams of omega-3s daily to lower triglycerides or one gram per day for patients who have been diagnosed with coronary heart disease. The AHA also recommends that individuals without diagnosed coronary heart disease eat oily fish and foods rich in alpha-linolenic acid (found in plants, particularly flaxseeds and flaxseed oil, chia seed and hemp seeds).

Flexibility

Omega-3s may also help improve joint health and flexibility. Improved flexibility means that you move and walk better. A major reason many people become less flexible with age is joint pain due to rheumatoid arthritis (RA) or osteoarthritis. Rheumatoid arthritis is related to inflammation of the joints.

Many people with RA who take omega-3 supplements report that they experience less joint pain and reduced morning stiffness. According to the National Center for Complementary and Alternative Medicine (NCCAM), omega-3 fatty acids prompt the body to produce anti-inflammatory compounds. A 2006 study published in the *American Journal of Clinical Nutrition* reports that omega-3s may also decrease the body's production of inflammatory molecules. In both of these ways, omega-3s are potent anti-inflammatory agents.

MEMORY

Essential fatty acids can also help you think more clearly and help improve your memory. Half of the brain is made up of healthy fatty acids, so the brain needs healthy fats to function properly. Deficiencies of EFAs can lead to abnormalities in brain structure.

Sufficient omega-3s may be important for preventing problems with cognitive function. A 2004 study published in the *Journal of Nutrition, Health and Aging* reported that omega-3s play an important role in preventing Alzheimer's disease. Alzheimer's disease—the sixth leading cause of death in the United States according to the Alzheimer's Association®—is a loss of cognitive ability that causes problems with memory and thinking.

The 2004 study reported that a deficiency of omega-3 fatty acids led to abnormalities in the brain. Supplementing the diet with DHA slowed accumulation of brain-clogging plaques and "tangles" associated with Alzheimer's disease. DHA also plays a role in the parts of the brain involved with forming new memories, and higher levels of DHA enhance memory and learning.

EYESIGHT

In addition to changing how you are seen, EFAs can also improve how you see! A fatty acid deficiency can lead to vision problems. DHA makes up around 60 percent of the fatty acids in the retina of the eye. Healthcare practitioners recommend that pregnant women take DHA supplements to support proper fetal vision (and brain) development. DHA can also support vision in adults. Sufficient fatty acids protect against two major causes of blindness in humans, *retinopathy* and *macular degeneration*. Retinopathy is impairment of the retina of the eye caused by damage to the blood vessels in the back of the eye. With macular degeneration, the tissue in the back of the retina deteriorates, causing blurring or a blind spot in the center of the field of vision.

A study published in 2001 in the *American Journal of Clinical Nutrition* studied over 4,000 women 50 years of age or older. At the time of the study, none of the women had been diagnosed with macular degeneration. Researchers reported that over the 10-year period of the study, women who consumed higher amounts of DHA had a lower risk of developing macular degeneration.

Moods

Finally, EFAs may help improve how you feel. Several studies indicate that EFAs can help with depression and bipolar symptoms. A 2007 study published in the *Journal of Clinical Psychiatry* reviewed clinical trials that used omega-3s to manage depression and mood disorders. The study's authors reported that omega-3s had a significant antidepressant effect, according to 10 double-blind, placebo-controlled studies.

Omega-3s may be particularly helpful in helping with depression connected with bipolar disorder. In a 2006 study published in the *British Journal of Psychiatry*, researchers found that over a 12-week study period, one gram of EPA per day alleviated depression symptoms in the individuals studied.

SOURCES OF HEALTHY FATTY ACIDS

Many dietary supplements can help you increase your intake of healthy fatty acids. Some of my favorites include:

Fish Oil. You can get healthy fatty acids from fish by eating fish or by taking fish oil supplements. Fish oils made from salmon, mackerel, herring and sardines may be the most beneficial, as these oils contain more omega-3s than other fish.

Krill Oil. Krill oil comes from krill, unique shrimp-like animals that live in the Antarctic Ocean and are the primary food for whales, penguins and other wildlife. Only a small percentage of krill is harvested for human consumption. Krill oil contains a small amount of astaxanthin, an antioxidant. Krill is a phospholipid, the type of fat that makes up your cell membranes and can pass the blood-brain barrier, meaning that it can nourish the brain. The body also absorbs phospholipids more easily than other types of fat.

Evening Primrose Oil. Evening primrose oil is pressed from seeds from the evening primrose, a plant with yellow flowers native to North America. The oil is particularly beneficial for women in menopause, partly because it is rich in GLA. One function of GLA is helping produce hormone-like molecules called *prostaglandins* that act as short-range messengers in the body. By helping increase prostaglandin production, evening primrose oil may counter menopause-related hormonal changes. It can also help maintain beautiful skin and may relieve hot flashes in some women.

Flaxseeds and Flaxseed Oil. Both flaxseeds and flaxseed oil are an excellent source of alpha-linolenic acid, and can help vegetarians get sufficient omega-3s. When taken internally, both flaxseeds and flaxseed oil can help with skin disorders such as psoriasis. The seeds also contain lignans, a class of phytoestrogens that may help with menopausal symptoms.

Chia Seeds. Chia seeds are tiny black or white seeds from the *Salvia hispanica* plant, which is native to Mexico and Central America. Chia seeds are one of the richest plant sources of omega-3 fatty acids. The seeds typically contain about 60–64 percent ALA.

Borage Oil. The borage flower (*Borago officinalis*), also known as the starflower, has blue flowers with five triangular petals. Borage oil comes from the seeds of the plant. It is rich in GLA and may help relieve pain and inflammation in the joints. Borage oil may be particularly useful for promoting healthy skin and nails.

No matter what source you choose, increasing your intake of these important fatty acids can help support a healthy heart, brain and joints!

Life is Short, Eat Chocolate

Everybody loves chocolate. And no wonder! Because chocolate tastes so good, eating it stimulates production of *endorphins*, chemical messengers that signal the brain to feel pleasure. Dark chocolate also has been linked to *serotonin*, an important neurotransmitter that acts as an antidepressant.

Besides making you feel good, chocolate can have many health benefits. In its purest form, chocolate (cocoa) is an antioxidant powerhouse. Blueberries, which are often touted as a superfood with amazing antioxidant abilities, don't hold a candle to dark chocolate! In terms of oxygen radical absorbance capacity (ORAC) units, developed to measure antioxidant potential by the United States Department of Agriculture (USDA), dark chocolate has 13,120 ORAC units per ounce, compared to 2,400 ORAC units per ounce for blueberries.

And the benefits don't stop there! Dark chocolate contains *phenols*, plant-based compounds that can help lower blood pressure. Another beneficial component of chocolate is *flavanols*, a class of plant compounds. Flavanols in chocolate include catechin and epicatechin, which also give health benefits to green tea.

Certain cultures in different parts of the world regularly consume cocoa, have very few diseases and live very long lives. For example, a 2006 article published in the *Journal of Cardiovascular Pharmacology* described the Kuna Indians of Panama. The Kuna Indians typically have low levels of cardiovascular disease and hypertension. However, when they migrate to urban areas and adopt urban diets, Kuna Indians develop cardiovascular disease at rates similar to the general population.

To determine what elements of their diets were protecting the Kuna Indians from cardiovascular problems, researchers compared the diets of Kuna Indians living in remote islands with Kuna Indians living in a suburb of Panama City. The researchers discovered that Kuna Indians who followed an indigenous diet typically consumed more than five cups of a traditional flavanol-rich cocoa drink daily, while urban dwellers ate little flavanol-rich cocoa. The researchers concluded that the Kuna's cocoa drink may play an important cardioprotective role.

Studies back up the health benefits of chocolate. A study published in 2008 in the *Journal of Nutrition* concluded that flavanols from chocolate may decrease the risk of developing cardiovascular disease. The study examined a group of men and women with impaired glucose tolerance, a precursor to diabetes that can also increase the risk of heart disease. The participants were divided into two groups. One group ate 100 grams of flavanol-rich dark chocolate daily while the other group ate 100 grams of white chocolate (white chocolate contains no cocoa paste, liquid or powder and therefore lacks the flavanols found in dark chocolate). The researchers found improvements in insulin sensitivity, and decreases in total cholesterol in the group that consumed dark chocolate.

But before you start gobbling down a candy bar, take note. To get chocolate's benefits, you need to consume dark chocolate—the darker the better! Eat chocolate with at least a 65 percent cocoa content, and watch out for extra ingredients that can reduce or even negate the benefits of chocolate. Many chocolate candy bars contain added butter and sugar, which add calories to chocolate and make it less healthful. Chocolate also commonly contains milk, which interferes with antioxidant absorption.

And remember: whatever its benefits, chocolate is not a calorie-free food. Don't eat a pound of it all at once! Portion control is extremely important. A bar of dark chocolate contains about 400 calories, so don't eat more than a half a bar a day. And on days you eat chocolate, reduce food intake by 200 calories so that your body weight does not increase. In the 2008 *Journal of Nutrition* study, participants were carefully instructed to reduce calorie intake to avoid weight gain.

MY MAGIC POTION

This amazing, delicious, antioxidant chocolate drink is great for circulation, energy and libido!

Ingredients:

Cocoa/cacao mixture:
    1 8-oz container of unsweetened cocoa or cacao powder
    10 tsp maca powder
    2 tsp cinnamon
    1 tsp turmeric
    1 tsp cayenne powder

Drink mix:
    1 Tbsp cocoa/cacao mixture
    3/4 cup water
    1/4 cup plain, vanilla or chocolate rice, almond or
      hazelnut milk

Directions:

Combine dry ingredients (cocoa/cacao, maca, cinnamon, turmeric and cayenne) in a large mixing bowl and stir until blended. This recipe will provide enough mix to make about 30 chocolate drinks. Store remaining powder in a cool, dry place.

To make the drink, add 1 tablespoon of the cocoa/cacao mixture to an 8 oz heat-resistant cup. Bring three-fourths cup water to a boil, add to cup and stir until dry ingredients are completely dissolved. Add plain, vanilla or chocolate rice, almond or hazelnut milk. Drink once or twice a day for a filling and satisfying beverage.

Make adjustments to the recipe as you find what you like. You can make this drink more or less spicy depending on how much cayenne pepper you add. You can also add more or less maca, depending on how it makes you feel.

We've already talked about the benefits of chocolate and maca, but all of the ingredients of my "magic potion" are extremely beneficial. I include turmeric to help improve circulation, cinnamon to support healthy blood pressure levels and cayenne to support proper circulation and brain function. All of these spices are incredible for supporting the immune system and keeping sickness away. That's why I call it my magic potion! (*Note: If you have high blood pressure, eliminate the maca powder.*)

Other Fountain of Youth Supplements

We've already discussed lifestyle and dietary changes that may help balance your hormones and fight diseases and aging. In addition to these changes, adding a few helpful nutritional supplements to your diet can make a huge difference to your health and happiness. Find your fountain of youth in the following nutrients:

MULTIVITAMIN

A multivitamin supplement can help remedy any deficiencies in your diet. A 2002 article in *Journal of the American Medical Association* noted that failing to consume optimal levels of vitamins increased the risk of developing diseases, including cardiovascular disease, cancer and osteoporosis. Vitamins support the immune system and regenerate skin, muscle, tissue, blood and bone.

In addition, by ensuring a more plentiful supply of vitamins and minerals, a multivitamin may also help you lose weight. A 2010 study published in the *International Journal of Obesity* examined the effects of multivitamin supplementation on 96 obese Chinese women between the ages of 18–55 years. Researchers divided the women into three groups and gave each woman a multivitamin, a calcium supplement or a placebo. The group that received the multivitamin lost an average of eight pounds over the 26-week study period. In addition, researchers noted that the women in the multivitamin group had improved cholesterol levels.

ESSENTIAL FATTY ACIDS (EFAs)

If I had to choose one of the best nutrients for overall health, it would be EFAs, often called "good fats." EFAs have antiviral properties and can help inhibit hot flashes, PMS, high cholesterol, inflammation, joint pain, skin problems and arthritis. EFAs can also support eye health, concentration and circulation.

As noted earlier, foods that are good sources of such "good fats" include oily fish (such as salmon, herring, mackerel, anchovies and sardines) flaxseed and chia seed. EFAs can be found either in capsules, gummies, chewables, liquid or even powder forms. Obtain EFAs from reliable companies that test their products to ensure they contain no PCBs (toxic chemicals that inhibit estrogen production and are linked to headaches, birth defects and skin sores), DDT (a pesticide linked to nausea, diarrhea and irritation of the eyes, nose or throat) or other environmental pollutants.

Astaxanthin

Activate your "longevity gene" with astaxanthin! This powerful antioxidant occurs naturally in certain plants and algae. As an antioxidant, astaxanthin may benefit the heart and immune system and fight inflammation. A study published in 2007 in the *International Journal for Vitamin and Nutrition Research* reported that when healthy, non-smoking males supplemented their diets with 4 mg of astaxanthin daily, levels of a type of fatty acid that encourages inflammation decreased significantly.

The body cannot synthesize astaxanthin, so you must obtain it from food or supplements. Animals that consume a diet rich in astaxanthin-containing algae, including krill, shrimp and wild salmon, are good sources of astaxanthin.

Vitamin D

Often called the "sunshine vitamin" because sunshine triggers its production in the body, vitamin D is crucial for many reasons. It promotes cardiovascular health; helps strengthen the immune system; and may help protect the body from osteoporosis, cancer, asthma, anxiety and many other harmful conditions. However, many of us are not getting enough of this vitamin from the sun—we spend a lot of time indoors and often wear sunscreen. The good news is that vitamin D is available in supplement form. I suggest taking 2,000–5,000 IU of vitamin D_3 (the supplement form of vitamin D) every day (See www.usda. gov, for recommended daily intakes.).

CoQ-10

We've already examined how CoQ-10 can benefit heart health. I consider CoQ-10 a must for several other health reasons, too. Why? CoQ-10 helps increase energy, because CoQ-10 is required for the body to produce ATP. Cells draw on ATP as their primary source of energy.

Every cell in the body contains CoQ-10. Organs that require a lot of energy to function properly—including the heart, liver, kidneys and brain—contain higher concentrations. CoQ-10 may help stimulate the immune system, boost endurance and defend the brain against diseases like Parkinson's disease and Alzheimer's disease.

GRAPES OF YOUTH

As mentioned earlier, another important dietary supplement is resveratrol. In addition to skin benefits, ongoing research indicates resveratrol has amazing anti-aging benefits. This information is not new—for years, researchers have talked about the benefits for the heart from drinking red wine. Some of the benefits of red wine come from resveratrol.

Given the alcohol content in red wine, it would certainly not be healthy to drink the amount of red wine needed to get positive effects. Taking resveratrol as a nutritional supplement, however, certainly helps! I believe that in the next few years even pharmaceutical companies may be producing products that contain resveratrol. Research suggests that in addition to enhancing heart health, resveratrol is also great for promoting more youthful skin, enhancing energy levels and reducing oxidative damage to cells. This is definitely a good dietary supplement to take!

ALPHA-LIPOIC ACID

This fatty acid is a supreme antioxidant. The body produces some alpha-lipoic acid, and absorbs some from food. With age, however, the body produces less alpha-lipoic acid. Some researchers suggest that supplementing the body's supply of alpha-lipoic acid may help fight aging.

Alpha-lipoic acid plays an important role in metabolism. When the body has a sufficient supply, it also functions as an antioxidant. It can fight inflammation, protect the nerves and ward off heart disease and Alzheimer's disease. A study published in 2007 in the *Journal of Neural Transmission* studied patients with mild to moderate dementia. For 12 months, researchers administered 600 mg of alpha-lipoic acid daily to individuals in the treatment group. They reported that this dosage slowed the progression of dementia in the patients studied.

Additionally, alpha-lipoic acid may help decrease insulin resistance in individuals with diabetes. When insulin resistance decreases, the body needs less insulin to process glucose, lessening the complications of diabetes. A 2006 study published in *Hormones* reported that 600 mg of alpha-lipoic acid taken twice daily significantly decreased insulin resistance in individuals with diabetes.

POMEGRANATE

A fruit native to the Middle East, pomegranate has many benefits for menopausal women. In addition to helping decrease hot flashes, pomegranate juice or supplements may help combat weight gain that often comes along with menopause. It may also help increase bone density, according to a 2004 study published in the *Journal of Ethnopharmacology*. The study found that administering pomegranate seed and juice extract to mice helped normalize bone loss in mice after their ovaries were removed, which induced menopause.

CRANBERRIES AND D-MANNOSE

Menopausal and post-menopausal women frequently suffer from urinary tract infections (UTIs). Such infections are caused by bacteria in the urinary tract and can produce a frequent need to urinate, pain during urination or cloudy urine. Up to 90 percent of UTIs are caused by *Escherichia coli* (*E. coli*). While healthcare practitioners often prescribe antibiotics to treat UTIs, a few herbal remedies offer possible alternatives.

Research suggests that cranberry juice may help prevent or treat UTIs. Cranberries contain proanthocyanidins, which can help prevent the bacteria that cause UTIs from sticking to the bladder walls. If the bacteria can't stick, an infection can't take hold. Try drinking 1–3 8-oz glasses of cranberry juice daily to combat UTI-causing bacteria, or one glass daily as a preventative measure. Look for a juice that is at least 27 percent cranberry juice that contains no added sugar.

D-mannose is another alternative treatment that may be helpful for treating UTIs. D-mannose is a simple sugar molecule found in fruits, including cranberries. Researchers say that it coats free floating *E. coli*, making it impossible for it to stick to bladder walls. If the *E. coli* does not stick to bladder walls, the body eliminates it, avoiding an infection.

Carpe Diem (Seize The Day)

I hope reading this book becomes more than just a guidebook, but redefines how you live each and every day of your life! Healthy and happy aging begins with good nutrition and supplements, balancing hormones (naturally, of course), exercise, reducing calorie intake and your attitude.

We live in a world of cause and effect and our attitudes have so much to do with our health. So, take a deep breath and exhale. Then take another deep breath and while you exhale, think: "I want to be healthy and I will begin now… seizing *this* moment." Just do it!

My Fabulous List

I once read that life should not be measured in the number of breaths you take but by the moments that take your breath away. Following are a few suggestions to make life more breath taking:

1. Buy a wig of a different color than your own hair, and go out to dinner. Wear it often.

2. Eat anything you want 10 percent of the time.

3. Write a story about yourself where the first sentence begins, "I can inspire others." Use your imagination and don't share the story with anyone.

4. Learn to breathe deeply. Deep breathing exercises are my favorite way to ward off stress and relax. (Deep breathing techniques are discussed on pages 39–40.)

5. Send or buy one red rose or favorite flower every week for yourself, so that it is the first thing you see when you open your eyes in the morning. Let it remind you that life can be beautiful.

6. Consider learning how to strip for your husband, lover or just yourself. Put some sexy music on and take off your clothes. I took a class at a school to learn how and I've never laughed so hard!

7. Take a magnesium bath once a week. Magnesium is fantastic for cleansing the toxins out of the body or just to relax.

8. Record your "oral history," or hire someone to help you record it. This history will remain as your immortality.

9. Be creative and learn to bake breads, cookies and cakes with unusual flours, such as almond, coconut and quinoa. It's fun and much healthier than baked goods from wheat and gluten.

10. (I saved the best for last!) Considering hiring a photographer and creating an album of yourself. Not nude—just sexy with props of beads, gloves, a hat, red satin sheets, high heels, etc. Just remember to smile and bring the perfume!

References

Appel L.J. "Effects of omega-3 fatty acids on cardiovascular health." *American Family Physician* 70, no. 1 (July 2004): 34–5.

Albarracin, C.A., B.C. Fuqua, et al. "Chromium picolinate and biotin combination improves glucose metabolism in treated, uncontrolled overweight to obese patients with type 2 diabetes." *Diabetes/Metabolism Reserach and Reviews* 24, no. 1 (2008): 41–51.

Andrade A.M., G.W. Greene GW and K.J. Melanson. "Eating slowly led to decreases in energy intake within meals in healthy women." *Journal of the American Dietetic Association* 108, no. 7 (July 2008): 1186–91.

Assunção M.L., H.S. Ferreira, et al. "Effects of dietary coconut oil on the biochemical and anthropometric profiles of women presenting abdominal obesity." *Lipids* 44, no. 7 (July 2009): 593–601.

Balbás G.M., M.S. Regaña, et al. "Study on the use of omega-3 fatty acids as a therapeutic supplement in treatment of psoriasis." *Clinical, Cosmetic and Investigational Dermatology* 4 (2011): 73–7.

Bastianett Covington M.B. "Omega-3 fatty acids." *American Family Physician* 70, no. 1 (July 2004): 133–40.

Farzaneh-Far R., J. Lin J, et al. "Association of marine omega-3 fatty acid levels with telomeric aging in patients with coronary heart disease." *Journal of the American Medical Association* 303, no. 3 (Jan. 2010): 250–7.

Fedorova I., A.R. Alvheim, et al. "Deficit in prepulse inhibition in mice caused by dietary n-3 fatty acid deficiency." *Behavioral Neuroscience* 123, no. 6 (Dec. 2009): 1218–25.

Fletcher R.H., K.M. Fairfield. "Vitamins for chronic disease prevention in adults: clinical applications." *Journal of the American Medical Association* 287, no. 23 (June 2002): 3127–9.

Fontana L. "The scientific basis of caloric restriction leading to longer life." *Current Opinion in Gastroenterology* 25, no. 2 (March 2009): 144–50.

Frangou S., M. Lewis M, P. McCrone. "Efficacy of ethyl-eicosapentaenoic acid in bipolar depression: randomised double-blind placebo-controlled study." *British Journal of Psychiatry* 188 (Jan. 2006): 46–50.

Georgiev, D., A. Goudev, et al. "Effects of an herbal medication containing bee products on menopausal symptoms and cardiovascular risk markers: results of a pilot open-uncontrolled trial." *Medscape General Medicine* 6, no. 5 (2004): 46.

Graham, J.M. (ed). *The Hive and the Honey Bee.* Chelsea, Michigan: Bookcrafters, 1993 (revised edition).

Grassi D., G. Desideri, et al. "Blood pressure is reduced and insulin sensitivity increased in glucose-intolerant, hypertensive subjects after 15 days of consuming high-polyphenol dark chocolate." *Journal of Nutrition* 138, no. 9 (Sept. 2008): 1671–6.

He K., K. Liu, et al. "Magnesium intake and incidence of metabolic syndrome among young adults." *Circulation* 113, no. 13 (April 2006): 1367–82.

Karppi J., T.H. Rissanen, et al. "Effects of astaxanthin supplementation on lipid peroxidation." *International Journal for Vitamin and Nutrition Research* 77, no. 1 (Jan. 2007): 3–11.

Kimura K., M. Ozeki M, et al. "L-Theanine reduces psychological and physiological stress responses." *Biological Psychology* 74, no. 1 (Jan. 2007): 39–45.

Kris-Etherton P.M., W.S. Harris, et al. "Fish consumption, fish oil, omega-3 fatty acids, and cardiovascular disease." *Arteriosclerosis Thrombosis, and Vascular Biology* 23, no. 2 (Feb. 2003): 20–30.

Li Y., C. Wang C, et al. "Effects of multivitamin and mineral supplementation on adiposity, energy expenditure and lipid profiles in obese Chinese women." *International Journal of Obesity* 34, no. 6 (June 2010): 1070–7.

Li, Q., A.H. Chen et al. "Analysis of glucose levels and the risk for coronary heart disease in elderly patients in Guangzhou Haizhu district." *Nan Fang Yi Ke Da Xue Xue Bao* 30, no. 6 (June 2010): 1275–8.

Lin P.Y., K.P. Su. "A meta-analytic review of double-blind, placebo-controlled trials of antidepressant efficacy of omega-3 fatty acids." *Journal of Clinical Psychiatry* 68, no. 7 (July 2007): 1056–61.

Lonn E., S. Yusuf, et al. "Homocysteine lowering with folic acid and B-vitamins in vascular disease." *New England Journal of Medicine* 354, no. 15 (April 2006): 1567–77.

McCullough M.L., K. Chevaux, et al. "Hypertension, the Kuna, and the epidemiology of flavanols." *Journal of Cardiovascular Pharmacology* 47, Suppl 2 (2006): S103–9.

Michnovicz J.J., H. Adlercreutz, et al. "Changes in levels of urinary estrogen metabolites after oral indole-3-carbinol treatment in humans." *Journal of the National Cancer Institute* 89, no. 10 (May 1997): 718–23.

Mori-Okamoto J., Y. Otawara-Hamamoto, et al. "Pomegranate extract improves a depressive state and bone properties in menopausal syndrome model ovariectomized mice." *Journal of Ethnopharmacology* 92, no. 1 (May 2004): 93–101.

Nakachi K., K. Suemasu K, et al. "Influence of drinking green tea on breast cancer malignancy among Japanese patients." *Japanese Journal of Cancer Research* 89, no. 3 (March 1998): 354–61.

National Institutes of Health. "Facts About Menopausal Hormone Therapy." June 2005. www.nhlbi.nih.gov/health/women/pht_facts.pdf.

Ndiaye M., C. Philippe, et al. "The grape antioxidant resveratrol for skin disorders: promise, prospects, and challenges." *Archives of Biochemistry and Biophysics* 508, no. 2 (April 2011): 164-70.

Ogden C.L., M.D. Carroll MD, et al. "Prevalence of overweight and obesity in the United States, 1999-2004." *Journal of the American Medical Association* 295, no. 13 (April 2006): 1549–55.

Omran H., D. McCarter D, et al. "D-ribose aids congestive heart failure patients." *Experimental and Clinical Cardiology* 9, no. 2 (2004):117–8.

Richter W.O. "Long-chain omega-3 fatty acids from fish reduce sudden cardiac death in patients with coronary heart disease." *European Journal of Medical Research* 8, no. 8 (Aug. 2003): 332–6.

Rizos I. "Three-year survival of patients with heart failure caused by dilated cardiomyopathy and L-carnitine administration." *American Heart Journal* 139, no. 2 Suppl. 2 (Feb. 2000): S120–3.

Schnyder G., M. Roffi, et al. "Effect of homocysteine-lowering therapy with folic acid, vitamin B12, and vitamin B6 on clinical outcome after percutaneous coronary intervention: the Swiss Heart study: a randomized controlled trial." *Journal of the American Medical Association* 288, no. 8 (Aug. 2002): 973–9.

Sinatra, Dr. Stephen T. *The Sinatra Solution: New Hope for Preventing and Treating Heart Disease.* Basic Health Publications, 2005.

Spasov A.A., G.K. Wikman, et al. "A double-blind, placebo-controlled pilot study of the stimulating and adaptogenic effect of *Rhodiola rosea* SHR-5 extract on the fatigue of students caused by stress during an examination period with a repeated low-dose regimen." *Phytomedicine* 7, no. 2 (April 2000): 85–9.

Stone, N.J. "Fish consumption, fish oil, lipids, and coronary heart disease." *Circulation* 94, no. 9 (Nov. 1996): 2337–40.

Tucker K.L., N. Qiao, et al. "High homocysteine and low B-vitamins predict cognitive decline in aging men: the Veterans Affairs Normative Aging Study." *American Journal of Clinical Nutrition* 82, no. 3 (Sept. 2005): 627–35.

Volker D., P. Fitzgerald, et al. "Efficacy of fish oil concentrate in the treatment of rheumatoid arthritis." *Journal of Rheumatology* 27, no. 10 (Oct. 2000): 234–6.

Yamaguchi, M., R. Hamamoto, et al. "Anabolic Effects of Bee Pollen *Cistus ladaniferus* extract on Bone Components in the Femoral-Diaphyseal and –Metaphyseal Tissues of Rats *in Vitro* and *in Vivo*." *Journal of Health Science* 52, no. 1 (2006): 43–9.

Index

Check out these other top-selling Woodland Health Series booklets:

Ask for them by title or ISBN at your neighborhood bookstore or health food store. Call Woodland at (800) 777-BOOK for the store nearest you.

Açaí Berry	978-1-58054-472-6
Antioxidants (2nd Edition)	978-1-58054-427-6
Aromatherapy and Essential Oils	978-1-58054-166-4
Arthritis and Joint Health	978-1-58054-407-8
Bee Pollen, Royal Jelly and Propolis (3rd Edition)	978-1-58054-174-9
Blood Pressure: A Naturopathic Approach	978-1-58054-107-7
Candida Albicans (3rd Edition)	978-1-58054-194-7
Chelation Therapy (3rd Edition)	978-1-58054-198-5
Chia Seed	978-1-58054-188-6
Cinnamon	978-1-58054-170-1
Coconut Oil	978-1-58054-464-1
Coenzyme Q10	978-1-58054-456-6
Colon Health (3rd Edition)	978-1-58054-197-8
Digestive Enzymes (3rd Edition)	978-1-58054-204-3
Digestive Health	978-1-58054-116-9
Fish Oil, Omega-3s and Essential Fatty Acids	978-1-58054-437-5
Flaxseed and Flaxseed Oil (3rd Edition)	978-1-58054-203-6
Grapefruit Seed Extract (3rd Edition)	978-1-58054-202-9
Green Tea: Matcha and More! (2nd Edition)	978-1-58054-215-9
Honey: Raw, Manuka, Tupelo and More!	978-1-58054-201-2
The Immune System (2nd Edition)	978-1-58054-164-0
Kombucha	978-1-58054-191-6
Liver Health	978-1-58054-397-2

Each booklet is approximately 32 pages and priced at $4.95.

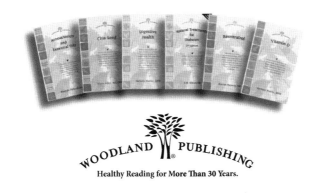

WOODLAND PUBLISHING

Healthy Reading for More Than 30 Years.

About the Author

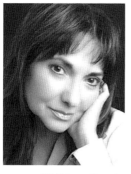

Roslyn Rogers, CNC, BCIM, has spent over 10 years traveling throughout the United States lecturing and giving seminars about health issues, including balancing women's hormones and pushing back the clock of aging naturally. Rogers is knowledgeable in a wide variety of health topics, including menopause, PMS, anti-aging, weight management, bone health, energy, healthy skin and dietary supplements. Rogers, 71 years young at the time of this printing, shows no signs of slowing down—evidence that she practices what she preaches.

Rogers has many years of experience in the natural health field, including 25 years in private practice as a Certified Nutritional Consultant (CNC) in New York. During this time, Rogers taught women about vitamins and herbs and refined her expertise in women's health issues. In addition to being a CNC, Roslyn is board certified in integrative medicine, a designation from the American Association of Integrative Medicine based on education, experience and training.

Rogers' lectures and seminars have positively impacted the lives of thousands of women. Rogers is known for her motivational skills as well as her sensitive and caring outlook on life.